Marital Therapy in Psychiatric Practice

An Overview

Marital Therapy in Psychiatric Practice
An Overview

Edited by
LINDEN F. FRELICK
and
EDWARD M. WARING

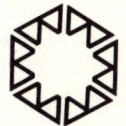

BRUNNER/MAZEL, *Publishers* • New York

Library of Congress Cataloging-in-Publication Data

Marital therapy in psychiatric practice.

  Based on a conference held at the University of
Western Ontario in London, Ont., Canada in June 1984.
  Includes bibliographies and index.
  1. Marital psychotherapy—Congresses. I. Frelick,
Linden F., 1938–   II. Waring, Edward M., 1944–
[DNLM: 1. Marital Therapy—congresses.   WM 55 M3432 1984]
RC488.5.M363 1987   616.89'156   86-20800
ISBN 0-87630-439-0

Copyright © 1987 by Linden F. Frelick and Edward M. Waring

Published by
BRUNNER/MAZEL, INC.
19 Union Square
New York, New York 10003

All rights reserved. No part of this book may be reproduced by any
process whatsoever without the written permission of the copyright owners.

MANUFACTURED IN THE UNITED STATES OF AMERICA

Contents

Contributors   vii

Preface   xi

1. Marital Therapy in Psychiatric Practice: An Overview   3
   Peter A. Martin

2. Indications for Marital Therapy   11
   Linden F. Frelick

3. The Initial Interview in Conjoint Therapy   30
   James E. Miles

4. Assessment of Motivation for Marital Therapy   56
   Michael Rosenbluth

5. Types of Marital Therapy in Psychiatric Practice   80
   Michael F. Myers

6. Marital Therapy: Outcome Research—Multiple Pathways to Progress   104
   Paul M. Cameron

7. Transference and Countertransference in Marital Therapy   136
   Herta A. Guttman

8. The Relationship of Sexual Therapy to Marital Therapy in Psychiatric Practice   165
   Edward M. Waring and Linden F. Frelick

vi   *Marital Therapy in Psychiatric Practice*

9. Combined Therapies   182
   Edward M. Waring

Index   207

Contributors

PRESENTERS

Paul M. Cameron, M.D., F.R.C.P. (C)
*Professor and Vice Chairman
Department of Psychiatry
Queens University
Kingston, Ontario*

Linden F. Frelick, M.D., F.R.C.P. (C)
*Associate Professor
Department of Psychiatry;
Associate Professor in Family Medicine
University of Western Ontario; and
Chief, Department of Psychiatry
Victoria Hospital
London, Ontario*

Herta A. Guttman, M.D., F.R.C.P. (C)
*Senior Psychiatrist and Director
Psychiatric Consultation Liaison Services
Sir Mortimer B. Davis–Jewish General Hospital; and
Associate Professor
McGill University
Montréal, Québec*

Peter A. Martin, M.D.
*Clinical Professor of Psychiatry
University of Michigan
Ann Arbor; and
Clinical Professor of Psychiatry
Wayne State University Medical School
Detroit, Michigan*

James E. Miles, M.D., D.P.M., F.R.C.P. (C)
Professor and Head
Department of Psychiatry
University of British Columbia
Vancouver, British Columbia

Michael F. Myers, M.D., F.R.C.P.(C), Dipl.A.B.P.N.
Coordinator, Medical Student Interns
Department of Psychiatry
Shaughnessy Hospital; and
Clinical Professor
Department of Psychiatry
University of British Columbia
Vancouver, British Columbia

Michael Rosenbluth, M.D., F.R.C.P. (C)
Assistant Professor
Department of Psychiatry
University of Toronto; and
Director of Clinical Services
Department of Psychiatry
Sunnybrook Hospital
Toronto, Ontario

Edward M. Waring, M.D., D.Psych., F.R.C.P. (C), F.A.B.P.N.
Professor, Department of Psychiatry
University of Western Ontario
London, Ontario

DISCUSSANTS

Reid Finlayson, M.D., F.A.B.P.N. (P), F.R.C.P. (C)
Associate Professor
Department of Psychiatry
University of Western Ontario
London, Ontario

Dermot Hurley, M.S.W., C.S.W.
Department of Child Psychiatry
Victoria Hospital
London, Ontario

Contributors

Ernest W. McCrank, M.D., F.R.C.P. (C)
Associate Professor and
Coordinator of Continuing Education
University of Western Ontario
London, Ontario

Susan J. O'Neil, M.S.W., C.S.W.
Social Work Manager
Department of Psychiatry
Victoria Hospital
London, Ontario

Paul G.R. Patterson, M.D., D.Ch.Psy., D.Psy., F.R.C.P. (C)
Associate Professor
Department of Psychiatry and Paediatrics
University of Western Ontario; and
Director, Child Psychiatry
Victoria Hospital
London, Ontario

Lila Russell, M.S.W., C.S.W.
Clinical Assistant Professor
Department of Psychiatry
University of Western Ontario; and
Co-Director of Human Sexuality Clinic
Victoria Hospital
London, Ontario

Preface

In June, 1984 a 2-day conference on marital therapy in psychiatric practice was held at The University of Western Ontario in London, Ontario, Canada. Psychiatrists who have previously published papers on marital therapy were invited to present overviews on eight topics crucial to practice:

1. Indications
2. Initial assessment
3. Evaluation of motivation
4. Type of marital therapy
5. Evaluation of outcome
6. Transference issues
7. Sex and marital therapy
8. The combination of marital therapy with other therapeutic modalities

Dr. Peter Martin, author of *A Marital Therapy Manual*, was invited to give an overview of marital therapy.

The presentations were organized to provide a formal discussion of each paper and dialogue between the conference participants, which was audiotaped. We have attempted to edit the book following this conference format. The presentation cannot convey the opportunities for informal discussion and personal interaction which conference organizers, presenters, discussants, and participants enjoyed.

Several comments about the motivations for organizing

the conference may be of interest to the reader. Marital therapy does not have a prominent place in the majority of psychiatric residency programs. The majority of practicing psychiatrists do not regularly do marital assessments, counseling, or therapy. We thought that publishing the proceedings of this conference might provide a reference book for residents and practicing psychiatrists as well as a stimulus for more interest in the topic. Second, the marriages of psychiatric patients have been a largely neglected area of academic interest. Recently, a series of papers has been published on this topic both in psychiatric and family practice journals and these papers are referenced. Finally, we believe the papers will be of interest to all mental health professionals and will provide stimulus to collaborative efforts to study the effectiveness, efficiency, and humaneness of marital therapy in specific patient populations.

We wish to acknowledge the significant contributions made to the success of the conference to the conference coordinator, M. Frelick, and the staff of the office of Continuing Medical Education at the University of Western Ontario, D. McCormick, D. Dalley, and J. Niles. We wish to acknowledge the assistance of S. Lowery, Clerical Supervisor, Department of Psychiatry, Victoria Hospital, South Street, and the secretarial support staff for their help with the transcription, typing, and preparation of this manuscript. We wish to acknowledge the support of the Eccles Fund, University of Western Ontario, the Royal College of Physicians and Surgeons, and the Pfizer Drug Company. Finally, we wish to express our appreciation to Brunner/Mazel for agreeing to publish the proceedings.

Marital Therapy in Psychiatric Practice

An Overview

Chapter 1

MARITAL THERAPY IN PSYCHIATRIC PRACTICE:
An Overview

Peter A. Martin

It is important that a speaker be in touch with the audience. We have all been members of audiences where the speaker droned on, unaware of the fact that he had lost his audience. We have listened all day to excellent scientific presentations. We seem to be in a relaxed, jovial mood, as an aftermath of a thought-provoking day. Given this state of mind, entertainment would be more in order than a ponderous talk entitled "Marital Therapy in Psychiatric Practice: An Overview." The topic is redundant anyhow since the 2 days of presentations will give you an excellent overview of marital therapy in psychiatric practice.

Therefore I am going to keep this introduction as light as possible.

I am reminded of a true story of an 8-year-old boy who fell through the ice on the lake and was drowning until his sister rescued him. He could hardly wait to get to school to tell his teacher of this important event. After he finished telling her and was waiting eagerly for her response, the over-burdened, overtired teacher looked up from her attendance book and said, "That's fine, dear, were you absent last Wednesday?" This became a password around his home. Whenever someone wasn't paying attention to a member of the family who was speaking, he or she would say to the inattentive one, "Were you absent last Wednesday?" If I ask, "Were you absent last Wednesday?", you'll know what I mean. Leaving our family and moving to psychiatry, I am reminded of the story of a patient who noted that the psychiatrist wasn't paying much attention to his tale of woe. In the same tone of voice, he said, "Yesterday I killed my wife with an axe," and continued on with no response from the overloaded therapist.

Perhaps, if I make this introduction anecdotal, make irreverent comments about a few sacred cows in the mental health field, throw in a few iconoclastic comments, it will help the reader to avoid "being absent" while reading the chapters which follow. In taking this approach I will also change the title from "An Overview" to "Personal Passions and Beliefs About Marital Therapy." Due to the experimenter effect on one's conclusions, it really will be the same paper, but my biases will be expressed openly instead of covertly during a supposedly objective review. There are many examples to illustrate that even research in the hard sciences leads to conclusions drawn from valid data which are selected out by the researcher to reach desired conclusions. These conclusions are often determined by important experiences in the early childhood of the researcher. Any data that would contradict the desired conclusions are ignored or discarded as invalid. This includes geniuses like Einstein who, after presenting his fantastic relativity theories said that he couldn't understand the work of his young colleagues at Princeton.

Another example from the mental health field exhibiting the researcher effect on one's work is the work of the late Margaret Mead. As a result of her research publications about growing up in Samoa, she became world famous. She reached a position where any new declaration of hers, no matter how unsupported or even bizarre, made newspaper headlines. Recently a respected anthropologist reviewed her work in Samoa and came to the conclusion that she had been taken in by the natives. They either told her what she wanted to hear or she selected out data that she needed to prove her preconceived conclusions. I see the same mechanism at work in the field of marital therapy. There are so many workers in the field operating from different theoretical and personal biases that confusion reigns. Those who follow the epistemologies-of-the-month brand of family therapy are so noisy about it (even though many are irrelevant to the consultation room), that a new term has been coined—"epistobabel." Scientists, whether in hard or soft sciences, are no different from the rest of mankind. Let me give you a few examples of possible differing conclusions based on the same data. Two women met on the street who had not seen each other for many years. One asked, "And how are your children?" "Oh," the other one answered, "Terrible! My son turned out to be a complete bum. He doesn't work, is on drugs and alcohol, and steals money from me. My daughter is not married, has two children, lives with me, and I have to raise them." Getting the picture, the first one asked, "If you had it to do all over, would you have any children?" To which the second woman replied, "Oh, yes, but not those two!"

As we read of exchanges between charismatic leaders in the field of marital and family therapy, I am reminded of a famous story of a furious argument between Lenin and Trotsky. Later at a big communist rally, Trotsky, to further his cause, triumphantly read a telegram that he received from Lenin. It said, "You were right. I was wrong.

I should apologize." As he waved the telegram in front of the audience, a man stood up and said: "That is not what the telegram says. It says, 'You were right. I was wrong. I should apologize?!!'"

In teaching marital therapy to psychiatric residents at my clinic at the University of Michigan, I try to remove personalities and countertransferences by saying: Listen to what the patient is saying. Collect the facts. Put the cards on the table and don't you read them. Let the cards read. If it is a pair of twos, let it read. Don't call it a full house or a lalapalooza. So the entire group auditing the presenter's supervision lets the cards read. It is simple; seeing is believing. However, when personal passions and beliefs get in the way believing becomes seeing.

What is important in this is that it all pertains to marital therapy. Marital partners bring into their marriages personal passions and beliefs that, like the scientists I have cited, cause them to select out those data that will lead to the conclusions they desire to reach. Marital therapy involves trying to remove transference reactions wherein attitudes and feelings that were bred toward parents in the past are projected onto present mates. The most common complaint that we hear in marital therapy is problems in communication. These problems occur because, given the same vignette, each mate will select out the data that lead to the sought-after conclusion and ignore other contradictory data. This is in sharp contrast to the way the marital partners reacted prior to marriage when they were in love. When they both looked at a beautiful sunset, saw the same thing and felt the same way about it, they were at one with each other—symbiotically bound. This was a state of being in love. People love other people who have in common with them seeing the same thing and feeling the same way about it at the same time. They don't even have to see what is really there but pick out the same data and deny the same data. For example, I asked a husband why he married his wife. He said that on their first date she invited him to her home for tea instead of forcing him to spend money on her. Then when she made both cups of tea using only one teabag, he knew he had found the right girl for him. At that instant they saw the same thing and felt the same way about it and fell in love. Of course, after the marriage she wasn't that careful about saving money and marital trouble began. The outstanding clinical example illustrating the same principle is a folie à deux. Here, husband and wife are so symbiotically bound that they share the same delusions and hallucinations. Now that's what you call close. They are the example par excellence of marital harmony and of love, but they had better stay at home and not come in contact with reality.

There is the story of the matchmaker who was called by a man in his mid-forties and told: "I want you to find me a wife. I haven't been married before because I am a perfectionist. I've had to have everything done perfectly and I am now ready to get a perfect wife. I want you to scout around until you find a woman who looks like a picture. Don't call back until you've found one who looks like a picture."

A week later the matchmaker phoned and gave our perfectionist the date, time, and address to visit his potential bride. He arrived at the door with flowers under his arm, rang the doorbell at exactly the right second and as the door opened, he saw a young woman with one slanted eye, a missing mouth and angular ears. Where there should have been curves, there were straight lines. He let out a shriek of terror, threw the flowers in the air and ran. After shaking for a week, he recovered enough to call the matchmaker at whom he screamed, "How could you do this to me? I told you explicitly that I wanted a woman who looked like a picture." To this, the matchmaker replied, "Well, either you like Picasso or you don't like Picasso."

Jay Haley is one of my favorite writers in the field of

marital and family therapy. He writes clearly and entertainingly. The fact that I often don't agree with the content and that he keeps changing gurus certainly should not be held against him. Many years ago he wrote that since we don't know what normal is for marriage, we don't know what to do in marital therapy. In rebuttal, in my book *A Marital Therapy Manual*,[1] I included research on psychopathologic marriages that fell into certain patterns. Following medical tradition which has derived normal values for human physiology after studying pathological functioning in patients, I derived normal values for marriage from studying psychopathologic marriage patterns. To this day, I use these normal values while doing initial diagnostic interviews for discovering what is wrong with the marriage and what will have to be done to bring the marriage into normal limits of marital functioning.

My current objection is to Jay Haley's recent statements about marital therapy. He is reported to have said that unlike family therapy which has come up with creative new theories and practices, marital therapists are to be criticized for coming up with nothing new but continuing to do marital therapy in the same way as they do individual therapy. He believes that the future of marital therapy depends on marital therapists coming up with a genuinely new approach. I have some difficulty in accepting Haley's comments since his present guru is the late Milton H. Erickson. Haley presents Erickson's ideas as a new approach in family therapy toward effecting change. The ideas presented are the same ones that I learned as a medical student from Dr. Erickson during the late thirties. Erickson was an artist at slipping around resistance to change by suggesting that it was the patient's wish to change and not Erickson's. Of course Erickson, contrary to most family therapists, had a deep respect for the power of the unconscious. He understood the ubiquitousness of ambivalence in human nature. Thus, so as not to be immobilized, for every position a person takes, the person has to push away an opposing wish. Erickson, by brilliant interventions, helped the person reverse the process by using the person's own buried wishes.

My position is that marital therapists are to be congratulated for being level-headed and seriously pursuing the field of psychotherapy without manifesting the faddish and religious fervor that leads to epistemological towers of Babel. I believe that the principles of psychotherapy are operating in all forms of psychotherapy whether they are recognized or not. There is no magic in techniques or in epistemologies. Technique is something that is used until the therapist arrives. Also, if there are three or more people present in a marital or family therapy session, one of them should know what reality is—preferably the therapist. I say this despite Carl Whitaker advocating the use of going crazy in doing family therapy. He goes crazy like a fox. If you want to call that going crazy, O.K., so it's crazy. However, caveat emptor! The character of the therapist is still one of the most important factors in all forms of psychotherapy.

For Haley to point to family therapy as a model to urge marital therapists to follow this lead is fascinating. Most observers agree that the field of therapy is in a phase of upheaval and confusion. In fact the term "epistemology" itself may have to be retired because so much confusion is associated with it. Let us hope that the disorganization reveals that family therapy is in a state of reorganization that will bring to it that dreaded word "homeostasis," a state that Haley finds objectionable.

Now, if I have upset or awakened anyone who wishes to object to what I have said, I already have an answer that is best relayed through the following story: The rabbi came home from the synagogue one evening looking more harassed than usual. His wife asked him what was wrong. He told her that he had been doing marital therapy all day and that was very upsetting to him. In the morning Mr. Cohen had come in and told him by the hour what a terrible, horrible wife he had. The rabbi's wife asked her harassed husband, "What did you tell him?" "Oh, I told him that he was right. Then Mrs. Cohen spent the afternoon telling me what a horrible husband she had." After a silence, the rabbi's wife asked, "What did you tell her?" "Oh, I told her that she was right." The rabbi's wife said, "You can't do that! You can't tell Mr. Cohen that he is right and then tell Mrs. Cohen that she is right." "You know," said the rabbi, "you're right."

REFERENCE

1. Martin, P.A. (1976). *A marital therapy manual.* New York: Brunner/Mazel.

Chapter 2

INDICATIONS FOR MARITAL THERAPY

Linden F. Frelick

Although interpersonal relationships are as old as Adam and Eve, and the marital relationship is social reality, much of our orientation in medicine has been on disease process and syndromes as they apply to individuals. The focus in traditional psychiatry has been no different. Psychiatry has been rooted in disease pathology and has focused on the intrapsychic dynamics of the individual. This medical model has a structural basis and we have focused on concepts of diagnosis, differential diagnosis, and indications and contraindications for treatment. This model is today preeminent in psychiatry in spite of the human tendency to live in the context of a marital union and a family constellation. The marital relationship and the family unit have been the basic building block of our society and have constituted the context for the development of the individual.

The recognition of interpersonal process and the marital and family system was initially understood by psychiatrists working mainly in child guidance clinics. They began the movement away from a strict focus on individual pathology and individual therapy.

The complexities of individual development were increasingly linked to and understood in the context of the interpersonal and family system. Initially this development was slow and did not center upon any unified theoretical framework or model. This pretheory stage was poorly defined and did not and could not fulfill the rigorous demands of the medical model. Thus marital therapy or systems therapy becomes a new orientation, with the patient being the system.

The coming together of two individual personalities creates a unique entity, the couple. When coupling takes place in the context of marriage we have the marital relationship. Thus we must conceptually consider three different factors simultaneously at work: complex intrapsychic factors (of the individuals), the interpersonal process (the interaction between the two individuals), and the marital process (the sociocultural context).

I have briefly discussed the intrapsychic process and its historical relationship to the medical model and would like to focus on some specific issues of the interpersonal process.

Hollender in discussing the interpersonal process proposed the concept of *dove-tailing*.[14] This notion addresses interacting needs between husband and wife which may make a marriage workable. These needs may be healthy or highly pathologic. Martin used the concept of the matching of needs to characterize the interpersonal process.[7,12] The matching is unique and the blending and matching of needs serves to characterize the relationship. Mismating occurs when the couple is not matched in terms of needs, when one mate outgrows the other, or where the partners' needs change. In general, the better matched the couple the more successful the marriage.

Goldberg also feels that successful interaction is less related to the degree of emotional health or pathology of the respective spouses than it is to the manner in which husband and wife fit together and are able to fill each other's needs, conscious and unconscious.[3]

Finally, our group at Victoria Hospital has looked at the concept of intimacy as an important process in interpersonal relationships and marriage.[4] The aspects of intimacy that we identified are affection, expressiveness, sexuality, cohesion, compatibility, autonomy, conflict, and identity. The more intimacy the fewer the conflicts in the relationship.

I will consider next the third factor, the "marriage" or the marital process. The notion of a healthy, ideal marriage has been based on the concept of two developmentally ready individuals forming a union that will serve and fulfill their individual needs and maximize personal growth in the life cycles and stages ahead. Its character is formed by expectations, needs (conscious and unconscious), social values, family expectations, economics, religion, and the fit of these individuals.

An idealized marriage is often the expectation of our society.[5] There is a set of expectations and these may be healthy or unhealthy. These expectations have to do with needs for love, affection, sex, companionship, communication, financial security, intimacy, and commitment.

Couples may wish to have children in an attempt to recapitulate the experience of their own family or to attain an idealized version of what they didn't have. Unfulfilled expectations are probably the most common problem. When expectations are mutually gratified, harmony exists.

It is probable that even the best of marriages go through difficult times. It is evident that marriage itself goes through a series of passages. These cycles and shifts are exceedingly important because they can act as crisis points and growth points. Indeed, we see couples in therapy at different moments in the life cycle. It is important to recognize that the process of the marital relationship varies over time.

Perhaps this is compounded at times by mismating, individual pathology, uneven growth, or unrealistic expectations in an idealized marriage. A pathologic relationship or mismating might include the use of marriage to escape a bad family situation, sexual attraction as the basis for marriage, neurotic needs, or insatiable needs for love.

To accentuate the clinical importance of this area the following findings are presented.

Sager et al. has noted that 50 percent of patients requesting psychotherapy did so largely due to marital difficulties.[10]

Gurin et al. found that marital concerns ranked first as the reasons that people seek help for emotional problems.[11]

Martin noted that it is at times difficult to make a distinction between marital and sexual therapy because 75 percent of the patients have had both problems.[7]

Since the vast majority of couples presenting are married, we will use the term "marital therapy." Although all the definitions of marital therapy relate to the interpersonal and marital process, it should be noted that individual therapy can have profound effects on the marital system. Consequently, I will describe a range of therapies from individual to combined therapies, all of which will represent approaches to the treatment of couples.

I will present a number of definitions of marital therapy and briefly mention some of the commonly described therapies.

Walrond-Skinner defines family therapy as the psychotherapeutic treatment of the family system.[9] He describes conjoint marital therapy as a subspecialty, which addresses itself to the specificity of the marital system.

Beavers uses the concept of couples therapy.[13] He defines couples therapy as a strategy in psychotherapy that arranges to intervene in a committed couples relationship. Such a couple may be the same sex or heterosexual, formerly married, or living together.

Krueger states that couples treatment is to treat the pathologic interacting of a couple in a long-term relationship who are in conflict involving one or more of several parameters, sexual, emotional, social, or economic.[1]

Sadock states that marital therapy is designed to modify psychologically the interaction of two married people who are in conflict with one another along one of a variety of parameters—social, emotional, sexual, or economic.[8]

The following is a brief description of types of therapies as presented in most textbooks, with those of Martin and Sadock being the best examples[7,8]:

1. Individual therapy.
2. Individual marital therapy.

    A. Concurrent Therapy where each partner is seen by the same therapist but at different times.
    B. Collaborative Therapy with a different therapist for each partner.

3. Consecutive marital therapy.
4. Conjoint marital therapy where both partners are seen together with one or two therapists.
5. Four-way therapy.
6. Group psychotherapy.
7. Combined therapy.

All the definitions of marital therapy clearly focus on the interpersonal (factor two) and the marital system (factor three). Individual therapy addresses factor one, the intrapsychic, but with a notion of growth with the goal of improving skills in factors two and three. Therapy of the individual type, although traditionally analytic, currently reflects a range of therapeutic modalities and this therapeutic evolution is also evident in the type of conjoint marital therapy. The many models of conjoint marital therapy include communications, behavioral, client centered, systems theory, psychoanalytic, strategic, structural, and cognitive therapy. In reviewing the literature it is clear that there is a more solid body of literature associated with individual therapy, individual marital therapy, and conjoint marital therapy. Consequently we have, although sparse and at times superficial, a body of literature on indications and contraindications. I have attempted to outline these from the literature and will present a compilation.

I would now like to focus on some of the specific therapies and specific indications and contraindications for each.

1. Individual therapy

    A. *Indications*

    (1) When it is felt an individualistic approach is necessary to assist the individual to develop.
    (2) When one spouse denies the existence of a problem.
    (3) When the problem is stated by one spouse to be entirely due to the other.
    (4) When one spouse refuses to see a therapist.
    (5) When privacy or confidentiality are essential in a disturbed marriage.
    (6) When the original mother-child symbiosis is being repeated in the marriage.

    B. *Contraindications*

    (1) When the marriage is severely disturbed with crisis or threatened abuse, suicide, murder, or psychosis. This requires intervention but also is not conducive to the relative quiet needed for introspection.

2. Individual marital therapy

    A. *Indications for concurrent therapy*

    (1) When an individualistic approach is necessary

Indications for Marital Therapy

      to assist each partner to develop the capacity to better cope with each other.

  (2) When the power struggle is such that one mate has overwhelmed the other.

  (3) When highlighting the interpersonal aspects of the relationship has become essential for treatment.

  (4) When one or both mates have the capacity for intrinsic exploration and change.

B. Contraindications

  (1) Severe psychosis.

  (2) A severe character disorder in one or both partners, excessive sibling rivalry, or jealousy, all of which prevents the partners from sharing the therapist.

  (3) Family secrets that can be exposed.

B. Indications for collaborative therapy

  (1) Where there is a secret that one mate does not want revealed.

  (2) When one mate does not want to be treated by the same therapist.

C. Contraindications

  (1) When one mate cannot tolerate not knowing what is going on in the other's therapy.

  (2) When the two therapists involved have difficulty in communicating or cannot stand supervision of their work.

3. Consecutive marital therapy

  A. Indications

  (1) When a disturbed marital equilibrium occurs resulting from the first mate's therapy, which leads to the second marital partner entering

therapy with the same therapist. When the completion of the first therapy has not resulted in the establishment of a homeostatic marriage and both partners wish the second mate to enter treatment with the same therapist to achieve this result.

B. Contraindications

(1) When either mate is opposed to the use of the same therapist
(2) When one mate is seeking divorce and the other believes that treatment will be for the purpose of perpetuating the marriage.

4. Conjoint marital therapy

A. Indications. These indications are compiled from a variety of authors including Frankel, Glick, Martin, Sadock, and Kessler.[2,6-8,12]

(1) When methods of individual therapy have failed to resolve the marital difficulties, or would be likely to fail because of insufficient motivation.
(2) When the onset of distress in one or both partners clearly relates to marital events.
(3) When marital therapy is requested by the members of the couple who are in conflict or unable to resolve conflict.
(4) When there are problems of communication between partners, for example, one spouse may be intimidated by the other, may react with anxiety when attempting to tell the other about thoughts or feelings, or may project onto the other unconscious expectations.
(5) When a problem is related to the series of complex interactions that when improperly carried out cause the marriage to deviate from the ideal. Thus conflicts may exist in one of several

Indications for Marital Therapy

areas, for example, sexual, or when there is difficulty in establishing satisfactory roles in the social, economic, parental, or emotional areas.

(6) When distortions are gross and when speed in halting marital disintegration is a critical factor.

(7) When problems involve acting out and are due to character disturbances.

(8) Sexual problems. In recent years conjoint treatment for sexual problems has shown increasing promise. Common sexual problems have often proven resistant to individual treatment. When these same problems are viewed in an interactional framework and treated with both partners present using a combination of sex therapy and marital therapy, results are surprisingly effect and rapid results have been obtained.

(9) When sexual therapy has failed due to a disturbed interpersonal relationship.

(10) When the child is the identifiable patient. Many couples are seen for therapy as a result of the child presenting as the identifiable patient.

(11) When distress or symptoms develop in one spouse as a result of therapy with the other.

(12) When the individual patient uses most of the individual psychotherapy session to talk about the other spouse.

(13) When couples are in the process of breaking up.

(14) When individual, group, or pharmacotherapy has failed due to the presence of destructive forces in the marriage.

B. Contraindications

(1) When there is clear evidence that the individual psychopathology rather than the marital interaction is the focus of the conflict.

(2) Where one spouse refuses to participate because of anxiety or fear.
(3) Where one or both parties absolutely wants to get a divorce or where one or more partners are uncommitted to work on the marriage.
(4) Where there is severe psychosis or paranoid elements in one or both marital partners; in this type of marriage homeostatic mechanisms are a protection against psychosis.
(5) Where there are secrets the marital partners don't want to reveal, such as infidelity or homosexuality.

It would not be appropriate to talk about indications and contraindications without recognizing that there is another view, which is addressed by Walrond-Skinner.[9] He makes the point that some therapists believe that a failure of any other treatment or any presenting problem is an indication for marital therapy. In fact, those holding this position would view the contraindications as indications and argue that it is the chosen modality of treatment or the skill of the therapist that is at fault. Simply put, this argument would state that not all couples are suited for a particular therapy. For example, those couples who perhaps are acting out and are not psychologically minded are not good candidates for analysis but might be appropriate for cognitive or behavioral marital therapy. This notion of matching patients to the therapy and the therapist is clearly important and requires more study.

It is increasingly being recognized that it is necessary to utilize a multidimensional or multiaxial approach, viewing the individual in the context of a relationship. In the context of a marital system, a broadly trained eclectic therapist will tailor a number of treatment modalities to the needs of the system. The alternative to this approach is to utilize a narrow theoretical framework with specific indications and specific approaches into which only those selected cases fit.

In summary, I have attempted to identify three important dimensions that contribute to the complexity of marital therapy; the intrapsychic, the interpersonal, and the marital system. These have been briefly described and the interaction and development of these three dimensions identified. The complex interaction of these variables can only be understood via a systems approach. The systems approach is still in its conceptual infancy. The indications for therapy require much more elaboration and clarification and I am confident that this will evolve with more research, clinical experience, and theoretical reconciliation.

REFERENCES

1. Krueger, D.W. (1979). Clinical considerations in the prescription of group, brief, long-term, and couples psychotherapy. *Psychiatric Quarterly,* 51(2), 92–105.
2. Frankel, S. (1977). An indication for conjoint treatment—An application based on the assessment of individual psychopathology. *Psychiatric Quarterly,* 49(2), 96–105.
3. Goldberg, M. (1982). The dynamics of marital interaction and marital conflict. *Psychiatric Clinics of North America,* 5(3), 449–467.
4. Waring, E.M., Tillman, M.P., Frelick, L., Russell, L., & Weisz, G. (1980). Concepts of intimacy in the general population. *The Journal of Nervous and Mental Disease,* 168(8), 471–474.
5. Grunebaum, H., & Christ, J. (Eds.). (1976). *Contemporary marriage, structure and dynamics and therapy.* Boston: Little Brown and Company.
6. Glick, I.D., & Kessler, D.R. (1980). *Marital and family therapy* (2nd ed.). New York: Grune and Stratton.
7. Martin, P. (1980). Marital therapy. In H.I. Kaplan, A.M. Freedman, B.J. Sadock (Eds.). *Comprehensive textbook of psychiatry III* (3rd ed.) (pp. 2225–2233). Baltimore: Williams and Wilkins.
8. Sadock, V.A. (1976). Marital therapy. In B.J. Sadock, H.I. Kaplan, & A.M. Freedman (Eds.). *The Sexual Experience* (pp. 496–504). Baltimore: Williams and Wilkins.
9. Walrond-Skinner, S. (1978). Indications and contra-indications for the use of family therapy. *Child Psychology and Psychiatry,* 19, 57–62.
10. Sager, C., Sundlick, R., Kremer, M., et al. (1968). The married in treatment. *Archives of General Psychiatry,* 19, 205–217.
11. Gurin, G., Veroff J., & Feld, S. (1968). *Americans view their mental*

health: *A nationwide interview survey.* Joint Commission on Mental Illness and Health Monograph, Series Four. New York: Basic Books.
12. Martin, P. (1976). *A marital therapy manual.* New York: Brunner/Mazel.
13. Beavers, W.R. (1982). Indications and contra-indications for couples therapy. *Psychiatric Clinics of North America,* 5(3), 469-478.
14. Hollender, M.H. (1959). Marriage and divorce. *Archives of General Psychiatry,* 1, 661-667.

DISCUSSION

Susan J. O'Neil, M.S.W. *(Victoria Hospital, London)*

Indications for marital therapy: What becomes clear is that the literature leaves us with a paucity of material on indications and contraindications in comparison with that available for the individual. This might suggest that marital therapy is still in an embryonic stage and that further input and study is necessary. Dr. Frelick's presentation reveals his philosophical bias in favor of the developmental and systems approach. The marital system is seen as an entity with various stages and cycles that is affected by the systems which form it, that is, the individual, and those systems around the individual. I feel this is an important concept that we must keep in mind as we see individuals and couples. This fact is emphasized in the paper as the three dimensions—of intrapsychic, interpersonal and the marital system—which are developed and examined. Another important theme is that of matching patients to the therapy and therapist. Dr. Frelick explores which end of the marital therapy continuum we choose to practice from, that is, the multidimensional approach with a broadly trained, eclectic therapist versus a narrow theoretical framework with specific indicators and a select number of cases. Marital therapy is complex, both as regards the nature of the system being treated and the system treating it. This, I think, gives us food for thought.

Question: I am surprised that you didn't say more about the impact of individual psychotherapy on the marriage. Could Dr. Frelick say whether he feels there is an optimal time at which marital therapy should begin during formal individual psychotherapy?

Dr. Frelick: I think your question as presented is an important one that really hasn't been addressed in the literature review that I have presented. Clinically we may go two ways. We start off seeing people in individual therapy and at some point something happens that suggests that we move toward a marital approach. At other times you start with marital therapy and you end up moving back to individual therapy. Personally I have my own idiosyncratic ways of evaluating that. I guess that most people who practice have their own indicators for doing that and there is nothing really very clear to help us in the literature. From a historical point of view, there is no question that many people have talked about individual therapy as having tremendous impact on the family system—the notion that if you change part of a system you change the whole system.

I think that is why individual therapy has been so important and is really viewed as a form of marital treatment. I don't know if I can very easily articulate the specific things that happen. Sometimes for me the issue is one of the readiness of the couple to make a commitment to the relationship and to marital therapy with me. I often see individuals whom I think are not ready to make that commitment or are not ready from a maturity point of view (they don't have enough ego strength) so there are a lot of factors that I think move you one way or another.

Question: Dr. Frelick, I wonder if you would comment briefly on the relationship of divorce counseling to marital therapy. It seems to me that on occasion they slide back and forth. On other occasions when you challenge these persons you feel they are leaning one way and then they sometimes decide to lean to the other side. I noticed at one point that you said that was a contraindication to do conjoint marital therapy if one or both people want a divorce?

Dr. Frelick: I think Peter Martin has addressed this issue very effectively and I'm sure he will speak to this point if we ask him. Basically, at one time a traditional view of marital therapy was to bring a marriage together and have it work and anything else really was not viewed as therapeutic or a constructive thing to do. I think that is a view of maybe 20 to 25 years ago.

Today, of course, we really are in quite a different ball game, and there is no question that we see people for separation counseling, we see all kinds of couples now. We have a number of homosexual couples here that are involved in therapy and we are doing everything under the sun in terms of couple therapy. I don't think it is marital therapy to look at people as separating but certainly it is couple therapy. I think that couple therapy and marital therapy have that distinction and it is an important one. I personally like the broader view and I am in favor of doing whatever you have to do with people who are in an interaction that is in difficulty, whether it is keeping them together or helping them to go their separate ways.

Dr. Peter Martin: I'll jump in at this point. The marital therapist is in conflict when starting to do marital therapy because there is a value system involved. Are you going to opt for the individual unit or are you going to opt for the social unit? That is what brings up the issue of divorce. Ideally both the individual's good and the social unit's good will come together. In reality there are often instances where the good of the individual comes second to the good of the social unit, or that of the marriage. If your background is that of psychoanalysis or individual therapy, you tend to have difficulty in watching the blocks to the development and growth of one individual because your value system has put the social unit of maintaining the marriage below that of growth and development of the individual.

There is certainly a point in some marriages where the individual would have to be in collusion with the folie à deux in order to stay in the marriage. It is a problem that you have to try and deal with in therapy with each couple. At this point are you going to opt for the social unit or are you going to opt for the individual's right to growth, development, and freedom? It is more difficult when children are involved. If you have a couple without children, that makes your personal biases and prejudices easier to express. I am sure we are all aware that in doing marital therapy our own personal biases, prejudices, our own family of origin, come into the picture as well as our own marriages. Those marital therapists who are having difficulty in their own marriages tend to get involved in the same way doing marital therapy. You always have to be careful not to be involved in transference reactions.

I would like to add a couple of new indications for marital therapy that have come up in my practice in the past few years that I haven't mentioned before. One indication is when you do marital therapy on the basis of a referral from an analyst who says, "The analysis has stopped functioning because there is so much trouble in the marriage and we can't go on, so please see the couple and do marital therapy so the analysis can continue." The other indication for marital therapy is where both husband and wife are in analysis and both analysts call and say, "Please see these individuals for marital therapy so that we can continue with the analysis." Now, the first type, where one mate is in analysis and then the couple is referred, has an interesting selection. In seeing these couples my experience is that about 50 percent of these couples, the analyst was accurate that the mate is impossible and perhaps psychotic and you have got to clear this up so that the other spouse can continue the analysis. In the other 50 percent of cases, he was totally fooled and projective identification had taken place. Everything that the analyst had said against the mate was the picture of himself, which the analyst hadn't picked up. This type can be referred back to the analyst; I would say this was projective identification and your patient was talking about you. As Dr. Frelick mentioned, in a state of conflict you can't do individual therapy without peace or introspection. When both partners are referred we run into a different problem. In marital therapy the only way I know of to undo the fighting that takes place is to concentrate on the individual analysis and ask the couple how come they are failing in their individual analysis. Many patients that we see now are character disorders (narcissistic personality, borderline) who may come for marital therapy. So what I have begun to do is character analysis with contract marital therapy because of referrals from analyses that have failed. When we have both mates present we start doing character analysis, so there is a new addition to the indications for marital therapy.

Question: I wonder if one couldn't say that it is impossible not to influence a marriage by doing individual therapy. If you are truly a systems-oriented person you are influencing the marriage and the question is in which direction and how. It seems to me that if you have two people in individual therapy that perhaps the best way to conceptualize it is that their homeostatic mechanisms have been disrupted both internally and, therefore, in their relationship. If you were to see them together you would want to know what has changed. What has changed to disturb the equilibrium and can help their growth further by establishing a new equilibrium, not the old one, but a new one? That would be the way that you would want to proceed if you were to see the couple together. You might frame it as a developmental consequence of individual therapy that may not necessarily be a failure, but rather a challenge.

Question: At no point have you described the technique of couples group therapy. Would you make any comments about that?

Dr. Frelick: There really isn't much about this in the literature. I personally don't practice it and I don't know whether somebody is going to address this later on. It isn't commonly practiced in a lot of areas. For marriages with long-standing marital discord where patterns of communication are egosyntonic, the impact of group therapy is that the spouses will learn new ways of communicating from other couples.

Question: I'd be interested to know what Dr. Martin might like to say on this because what led me to my question were his comments about character analysis. It is my impression that group psychotherapy for individuals is fairly effective treatment with character disorders; I wonder if he would like to make any comments about that in connection with couples group therapy.

Dr. Martin: Couples group therapy has the highest percentage of good results when compared to other types of marital therapy. One of the reasons for this is that group therapy has the capacity for helping people with narcissistic disorders that individual therapy doesn't have. Couples groups are successful because things that we as individual therapists wouldn't dare to say to the patient, they don't mind saying to each other.

Dr. Cameron: I have a question about training. Both Susan O'Neil and Dr. Frelick made reference about the options of a therapist using multiple models or techniques or having specific populations of couples being referred for specific treatments. I have always been brought up in the tradition that eclectism and multiple models are important, particularly for a psychiatrist who may often be making the initial assessment. But the question is: Do you really see training programs where therapists learn multiple models, or do you see the therapist move toward certain models. Therefore, wouldn't it be better to have people working in groups? I wonder how your group has resolved that problem.

Dr. Frelick: I think that our group is very similar to what goes on in many, many places. It has a tendency to be somewhat idiosyncratic. We have talked for years and years about developing a focus and a conceptual framework for training for family and marital therapy in this center. It has been an incredibly difficult thing to pull together and I suspect that that is really the problem in many teaching facilities. What tends to happen is that there are certain personalities that emerge with certain types of orientation and then a kind of a school develops around them, like Minuchin in Philadelphia. Really, there is no good classically trained program that you can transport from place to place and is agreed upon by everybody. In my experience it is nonexistent and so what happens is that everybody picks up a bit of training here and a bit of training there and blends something and ends up with on-the-job learning, trial and error learning. I think that is where the state of the art is.

Question: One thing that would concern me is the suggestion that one should enter individual therapy with one member of a marriage about a marriage problem. I think that it takes a very skillful therapist not to get caught up in countertransference problems. I think that marriage is almost a contraindication to intensive individual therapy until both partners are included in the decision to go ahead with therapy. I think that if somebody wants individual therapy about a marriage problem, that one should be very careful.

Comment: I certainly don't agree with that at all and

would like to draw attention to what Dr. Martin said before. It becomes a question of where you place the value, on the marriage or the individual. There are cases where the individual is being destroyed by a bad relationship and comes for individual therapy. One is concerned about extricating that person from the destructive relationship they are in. The primary aim may be to destroy the relationship that is based on a terrible neurosis.

Dr. Martin: I disagree with that statement. Marital therapy is a frame of mind and the way you look at things. In doing individual analysis, having done marital therapy, I am a better analyst for that outlook and knowing what is going on in the marriage. In doing individual therapy analysis you are not aware of what is going on in the marriage and you are not concerned for the children—you are doing a very limited analysis.

Chapter 3

THE INITIAL INTERVIEW IN CONJOINT THERAPY

James E. Miles

I do conjoint therapy and I feel very privileged. To help relieve the misery and suffering that are the inevitable consequences of marital conflict is a very gratifying experience. As a child I wanted to be an explorer—perhaps journey up the headwaters of the Amazon—but unfortunately I am not overly endowed with physical courage. Conjoint therapy satisfies all my desires for exploration and, although not without risks, at least there are no crocodiles.

I have been seeing couples, referred as couples, for the past 15 years. Some characteristics of my patient population, from a review of 50 consecutive couples, are outlined in Table 1.

TABLE 1

	Age (years) Males	Females
Mean (SD)	37.9 (8.73)	35.4 (8.64)
Range	25–57	25–58

Marital Status at Assessment

Married	46 couples
Common-law	1 couple
Separated	3 couples

Duration of Current Relationship

Mean duration	11.26 years (SD = 8.94)
Range	1.50–30 years

No. Previous Marriages

	Married Once previously	Twice previously
Husbands	10	1
Wives	12	0

No. Couples with Children[a]

Mean no. children per couple	2.6 (SD = 1.18)
Mean age of children (years)	13.2 (SD = 8.28)

Abbreviations: SD, standard deviation.
[a] Thirty-seven couples.

The couples are seen conjointly one hour each week for an average of 12 visits. My aversion for individual sessions has been well expressed by Framo:

> I have found that the advantages of individual sessions (learning about secrets, for instance) are not worth the suspicions of the absent spouse and the conflicts of loyalty and confidentiality in the therapist that such sessions give rise to. Besides, each married person exists in the context of an intimate relationship, and breaking the couple into private sessions negates the context and obscures the collusiveness that goes on between married partners. I have learned that when spouses work on their intrapsychic conflicts in the presence of their partners, the latter develop a more empathic view of the spouse, especially when they come to recognize what their partners have had to struggle with during their lives. The dilution of the transference to the therapist I see as a plus in marital therapy; in more recent years, I have found it more productive to deal with the transferences of spouses to each other.[1]

The term "marital therapy" is, I think, misleading. It implies that the primary focus of therapy is the marriage. What is really occurring, however, is the psychotherapy of two individuals within, and enhanced by, the intense context of an adult's most important relationship. Conjoint therapy seems to me a much more accurate description of what actually occurs and in no way diminishes the importance of the transactional phenomena.

THE INITIAL INTERVIEW

In this section I will describe concretely what I do in the initial interview and the rationale. I have usually had no previous contact with the couple presenting for the first conjoint visit. They will have been referred by their family physician, often on the recommendation of a couple I have treated previously. This type of recommendation, although it may unrealistically enhance expectancy, is on balance a positive factor in that it helps to increase trust in the therapist, which is an important component in the development of a good patient–therapist relationship. Rarely, the referral will come with a letter from the referring physician. Most commonly, a minimal amount of information is obtained from the referring physician, or the nurse, by my secretary. I am not unhappy about the paucity of information prior to the initial visit, although I will request information from previous therapists subsequently. In my experience, the prior information is often misleading and can induce a bias that I then have to correct. Prospective couples are placed on a waiting list, and the time from first contact to first visit may vary between three and eight months. I am uncomfortable with the delay, although it surprises me that there are very few separations during this waiting period, even in very tenuous relationships.

When the couple arrives, I get them from the waiting room, introducing myself in the process. I seat them in two chairs facing mine, placed close enough together so that I can observe both of them simultaneously, and not have to flick my eyes from one to another like a spectator at a ping-pong game.

Prior to the initial contact with a new couple I experience a few minutes of anticipatory excitement mingled with anxiety. Despite broad similarities in the patterns of marital pathology, each couple presents a unique experience and challenge. The couple and I, from the first encounter in the waiting room, are engaged in mutual appraisal. For my part, I am sensitive to their appearance, age, dress, and behavior with each other as I see them in the waiting room and entering my office. I am particularly conscious of any incongruities in their appearance as a couple: Do they seem to "fit" together as a couple or, for example, is the husband immaculately and expensively dressed while the wife is dressed tastelessly, perhaps chewing gum and with her hair in curlers?

I am an active, open, and direct therapist with a standard interviewing format for the assessment phase. With the patients seated, and following some brief pleasantry to diminish the tension, perhaps some humorous comment on the problem of finding parking space or the difficulty in locating my office, I then ask them the following questions:

1. To each in turn, age and occupation.
2. To both of them (to see who takes the initiative to answer), the duration of the marriage, whether they had lived common-law prior to marriage, and the duration of the courtship.
3. To each in turn, whether they have been previously married and if so, to whom, the duration, and whether there were children of that union. If there were children, what are their names and ages, with whom do they live, and the nature of the individual's relationship with each child.
4. Where do you live? Is it a house, an apartment? Do you own or rent?
5. Who else lives in the house? Where there are children, their names, ages, physical, and mental health, and whether they are "good news" or "bad news" to each of the spouses. If there are other relatives, nannies, maids, etc., who they are, their ages, and how are they perceived by each of the partners.

At this point, perhaps five to 15 minutes into the interview, I have a considerable amount of information from observation of their behavior with each other and myself, as well as their answers to these straightforward questions.

In response to my initial pleasantry, is there any evidence of a sense of humor, a very important quality in terms of prognosis? Who takes the initiative? How does the other partner respond to this? Do they disagree with each other over, for example, the duration of the courtship, one insisting it was a year, the other 13 months? If one or both partners have been married previously, the therapist will have gained some appreciation of the significance of these former spouses and the children to each of the partners. Asking about the children reveals whether they are a "conflict-free" area where both parents are in agreement on child-rearing, or whether one or more of the children have become pawns in the marital conflict. These initial five question areas permit the therapist to get to know something about the couple and allow them to reassure themselves that they have a place in the world—a home, occupation, children—which is helpful when they are on unfamiliar territory engaged in an unknown and very anxiety-provoking experience.

Question 6 is, "Whose idea was it to come for conjoint therapy, and when did you first seriously consider it?" In a retrospective look at 50 consecutive couples, the wife had taken the initiative in 29 couples, the husband in nine, and nine were defined as mutual (with three unspecified).

This is a very useful time to make a direct inquiry about motivation by asking how each partner feels about undertaking conjoint therapy. The motivation of each partner is a central issue, and is a curiously neglected area in the literature.

> While one or both members of the dyad may have "low" motivation for working towards a happier and more functional marriage, they may have, in fact, very powerful alternative motivations for seeing a therapist.... When the lack of congruence between the goals of the therapist and one or both marital partners goes unrecognized, effective therapy may be seriously prejudiced.[2]

I categorized some of these alternative motivations[2] as:

1. *"We (I) have tried everything, now we can separate."* Here, one or both partners have already made a secret decision to separate, but are highly motivated to see a

therapist to assuage their guilt feelings by being able to state, "We (I) tried everything."

2. *"I'll get you, you bastard."* Typically in this situation, conjoint therapy is sought as just one more "battleground" in a protracted war waged relentlessly by a "warm and loving" wife against her "cold, unfeeling" husband. The psychiatrist's office, where affect is sanctioned and rewarded, is a particularly punitive locale for these husbands.

3. *"You look after her (him)."* In this situation, the primary motivation of one spouse is not only to get out of the marriage, but to ensure that the partner, who is perceived as "vulnerable and pathetic" has someone else to care for her (him).

4. *"Marital therapy as a career."* This rather rare motivation relates to couples who have been in virtually continual marital therapy with a succession of frustrated therapists since the early years of the marriage. In the author's experience, it most commonly occurs where the partners have married in response to strong familial or cultural pressures. The therapists serve as parental or societal symbols and the paramount motivation is to punish the therapist for the fact that they are married at all.

5. *"Obviously, I'm the innocent party."* In this presentation, the primary tactic is "blaming" and the partners are motivated to seek conjoint therapy to have their innocence confirmed by an authority.

6. *"Taking the heat off."* In this situation, one spouse has acceded to the other's demand for conjoint therapy by agreeing to attend while quietly harboring strong feelings of resentment and resistance. If it can be made explicit in the initial interview, a negative set about conjoint therapy by one partner can usually be dealt with readily. When, however, a negative set is denied and the reluctant partner

is attending with the primary motivation of alleviating pressure from the other partner, therapy is difficult.

7. *"Let's get out without fighting."* In this presentation, the primary motivation is not only to get out of the marriage, but most importantly to do so without open conflict—a pattern that has usually been characteristic of the marriage.

It is important that these other motivations be ever-present in the therapist's mind, especially during the initial contacts with the couple. If, in asking the partner of the initiating spouse how they feel about coming for therapy, a husband, for example, says, "I don't mind," one is immediately suspicious that he has agreed to come primarily to "take the heat off."

Question 7 refers to previous marital therapy, who with, when, the frequency of visits, the duration and each individual's perception of the outcome. Surprisingly often, one will give a positive report of the outcome, the other a very negative review, indicating a probable failure on the part of the therapist to have established a symmetrical relationship with the couple.[3] Some support for this perception is given by the fact that commonly these previous interventions have been individual visits for both, usually more for the wife, and most commonly they have only been seen conjointly on one or two occasions.

In question 8, I ask each partner for a brief statement of what they see as the problem in the relationship and its duration. Many couples will agree about the approximate duration of their conflict, but wide divergences are not uncommon. An extreme example of this is where the wife says there has been a major marital problem for 10 years, and the husband flatly denies that from his perspective there is any problem whatsoever. Asking for a brief statement of the problem is helpful in determining the degree to which each partner is prepared to take some share of the responsibility for their unhappy marriage.

This ranges from the unrealistic (and narcissistic) acceptance of 100% of the responsibility by one partner, to a complete denial of any responsibility by one or both partners, and attributing the "blame" entirely to the spouse.

Question 9 asks each partner what their expectations are of therapy. This helps to clarify each individual's goals and provides an opportunity to assess the congruence of their expectations. Where the wife states, "We would be able to talk better, and we could both change our behavior," and the husband says, "I'd like our relationship to be better, and I'd like to get over a number of resentments that I have," and if a more detailed inquiry of these statements supports their main thrust, one could tentatively conclude that there is some similarity of expectation and some sense of shared responsibility. Motivational issues may emerge strongly here. A partner who says, "I'd like to understand what went wrong so, just in case this marriage doesn't work out, I won't make the same mistake again," is probably signaling minimal motivation toward maintenance of the marriage.

Question 10 is phrased as follows: "May God strike me dead, I am not suggesting this at all, I just want to know what your thoughts have been: Why don't you pack it in?" The answers can be a rich lode of information, not only about the partners' previous and current impulses to separate, hence constituting another monitor on their motivation, but also about their reasons for not wanting to separate. Themes of love and commitment may easily emerge here or, conversely, their absence, and concerns may be expressed that have less to do with the relationship and more to do with the partners' apprehension over the practical and emotional consequences of separation and divorce.

Another value of this question is to allay anxiety. A common fear of people contemplating conjoint therapy is that the process will end in divorce. Raising the issue directly and early is, in my experience, helpful.

Question 11 is a sequence of three questions to each spouse. It is not clear to me how I choose the spouse to ask first, although often I seem to choose the partner who has spoken least. First, I ask, "How is your wife/husband a pain in the ass to live with?" I am not happy with this expression but one needs, particularly with couples who are extremely uncomfortable with conflict, to affectively sanction the expression of negative thoughts and feelings. Table 2, taken from a chart review of 50 consecutive couples, categorizes the 12 most common complaints that partners make about their spouses. The statements range from a total character assassination of the partner, for example, "He's a sexual flop" or "He has absolutely no integrity," to the even more ominous, "She's the sweetest wife in the world, she's absolutely perfect."

Second in this sequence is, "What is the good news about your wife/husband?" This provides an opportunity to focus on and assess the assets of the marriage. This is usually quite touching for the recipient of the good news, and such comments as, "Why, you've never told me that before" in a tone of pleased surprise are common. Sometimes the "bad news" intrudes into the "good news," as seen in such comments as, "I *used to feel* she was open and honest." On rare occasions, in marriages in extremis, there is a paucity of good news or what is given is invalidated by the manner in which it is presented. This usually has motivational and prognostic implications.

The third question in this sequence is phrased, "I want to make it absolutely clear that I am not attributing to you any Machiavellian intent, that is, I am not accusing you of plotting how to drive your husband/wife around the bend, but *how do you get even* with this person whom you find so difficult? What behaviors of yours do you know distress your spouse?" This question accomplishes a number of things: First, it is an indication of the person's degree of comfort with hostile feelings. Some individuals will reply, "Doctor, I'd never try to get even; I'm not that

TABLE 2
Complaints About Spouses (n = 50 Couples)

Wife's Complaints	Frequency	Husband's Complaints	Frequency
He doesn't talk to me	20	Poor Housekeeper	14
He criticizes me	20	She won't talk to me	13
Domineering	17	Unsatisfactory sex life	12
Doesn't care enough	15	Moody	12
Unsatisfactory sex life	12	Bossy	10
Bad Temper/ Angry outbursts	12	Nags	9
Drinks too much	8	Perfectionistic	8
Can't be counted on	8	She criticizes me	7
Insecure	8	Insecure	6
He doesn't listen to me	8	Stubborn	6
Unassertive/ dependent	8	Cold	5
Withdraws	6	Screams at the kids	5
Other	60	Other	73
Total no. complaints:	202		180

sort of person." Secondly, it allows people to openly acknowledge that they are fully aware of the specific behaviors that antagonize their spouse and in so doing, they are taking responsibility for what they do. The responses are often surprising, for example, a wife replied to the question, "I don't talk . . . that really gets him. I used to have temper tantrums and throw things, but I found that not talking is a lot more upsetting to him." Or a very obsessional husband who had stated as the "bad news" about his wife, "She doesn't pay attention to details. I work out plans and procedures for her for the efficient operation of the kitchen and she ignores them." This is guerrilla warfare of a high order. He delighted me, however, when asked how he got even, by replying, "I get very analytical and preoccupied with details; I tend to be too logical."

Finally, this question introduces or reinforces the fact that the couple are at war—full-scale war—and it is remarkably salutary, in my experience, to point that out to them. Most couples are well aware that they are miserably unhappy, usually blaming it on the spouse, but genuinely find it surprising to fully appreciate the complexity, pervasiveness, and intensity of their struggle with each other. As can be seen in Table 3, withdrawal is the most common method of retaliation for both sexes, comprising over a third of the wives' and two thirds of the husbands' revenge armamentarium.

The mean time for the foregoing interview format is

TABLE 3
Wife's Methods of Retaliation Against Husband (n = 50)

	Frequency
Withdraws	22
Nags	13
Fights/yells/outbursts	6
Withholds sex	4
Spends too much money	3

Husband's Methods of Retaliation Against Wife (n = 50)

	Frequency
Withdraws	28
Angry outbursts	3
Withholds sex	2
Does wife's chores	2
Has an affair	2

about 50 minutes, although with good rapport and a responsive, psychologically minded couple I have done it in 30 minutes. In the latter case, I would then start on a psychiatric history of one member of the dyad. In any event, I leave the last 10 minutes of the hour for an explanation to the couple of the following:

1. The theoretical model I use. This is based on Segraves's[4] theoretical outline, which I have found to be most congruent with my own experience. This theoretical structure is summarized as follows:

1. Because of the complexity and quantity of interpersonal stimuli and the limited information-processing capacity of the human nervous system, human beings develop cognitive schemas or templates to organize their interpersonal perceptions. These schemas influence the manner in which new information about people is perceived and assimilated.
2. It is hypothesized that in cases of chronic marital discord, both spouses have schemas for the perception of the mate that are both negative and markedly discrepant with the mate's personality. Clinically, this will be observed as a *fixed* misperception of the mate's character.
3. It is hypothesized that these schemas or tendencies toward misperceptions were learned from previous intimate experiences. The most powerful influences in the creation of these schemas are childhood experiences with one's parents, although they may be modified, for better or for worse, by later life experiences.
4. In cases of chronic marital discord, the person has difficulty observing differences between the external reality of the present partner and internal images or cognitive schemas for the opposite sex.
5. These distorted perceptions contribute to interactional sequences that maintain these distortions.

6. Repetitive observation of spouse behavior discrepant with the internal model for the spouse will result in a change in the representational model.
7. As this framework implies that perception of the spouse at any given moment is partially a function of the actual behavior of the spouse and partially a function of the representation model evoked, the degree of influence of the representational model on perception is a function of the ambiguity of the perceived situation. This implies that the use of clear and explicit communication patterns between spouses should minimize the amount of distortion possible.

I tell the spouses that couples in serious marital difficulty have usually had childhood experiences with parents that have made them wary of intimacy, and that have given them a distorted view of their partner. I briefly discuss the collusive nature of marital discord and illustrate it, depending on the degree of rapport, with an example from their own behavior during the session. If the rapport is not that good, I would use, at this point, an anecdote to illustrate collusion. I believe an explanation of the therapist's theoretical model is mandatory, and anxiety is reduced in the couple when they have an approximate flight plan. I further explain that I will be taking a psychiatric history from each of them in the next one to two sessions, which will complete the assessment period.

2. I offer at this point, although stressing that the assessment is incomplete pending their individual histories, a brief, *tentative* impression of the marriage. I reinforce such themes as the hostility that exists between the spouses and the indirect nature of its expression, their often high level of functioning in other areas of life except in intimacy, collusiveness, taking responsibility for one's behavior, and the importance of motivation. If there are realistic grounds for expecting that this couple will be able to do

well, I instill hope by communicating my sense of optimism, citing specific observations from the initial interview to support this, for example, sense of humor, pre-existing good level of marital functioning, and good motivation.

3. I make clear that I will not see them individually (with an exception I will outline later) and that I do not want telephone calls. To permit telephone calls is to invite unilateral material that would be much more usefully proffered in the sessions, and also threatens symmetry.[3]

4. I mention that the average number of visits is 12, but it varies considerably, and that termination is up to the couple. This latter procedure has worked very well for me and I have never had the slightest problem with it. Stating the mean number of visits gives the couple an approximate idea of the time involved, and also may function as a stimulus for them to work more actively.

5. Finally, I ask if the couple have any questions; I then thank them and indicate I would be willing to continue to see them, stressing that the decision is theirs.

At the end of the first interview, what has happened? Optimally, the beginnings of a good patient–therapist relationship, a reflection of the therapist's interest and empathy and the patients' trust and motivation. There will have been a release of tension by the catharsis, the instillation of hope, and perhaps the realization that the hour's experience was better than the couple fearfully anticipated. They will have felt that whatever took place in the session was within the context of emotional support from the therapist. The couple will have an approximate idea of what is going to take place in therapy and why it is going to take place. They may have accepted that they are at war, begun to see some of the subtleties of their combat, and may have started to examine more seriously their own role in the marital transaction.

I have a great respect for the vast majority of people who seek help for their floundering marriages. Marriage is the last bastion of privacy and I think it takes courage to face up to the fact that one is in difficulty, and to share one's marital secrets with a total stranger.

At the end of this initial interview, the therapist should have an idea of each partner's life situation, value system, social competence, as well as how articulate they are and their psychological-mindedness. The therapist should have some appreciation of the maturity of the individuals' defense mechanisms and some idea of their self-esteem and autonomy. The therapist should also have some sense of how committed the spouses are to each other, the level of their motivation, how they deal with conflict, and the pattern of marital pathology.

The therapist may also have some sense of the prognosis; this should not be too firmly held since, in my experience, initial impressions can be misleading and couples who look promising initially sometimes go nowhere, whereas couples who present a seemingly insoluble dilemma can do gratifyingly well.

VARIATIONS ON THE INITIAL INTERVIEW

The initial interview format as outlined above is appropriate for the majority of couples who present. Obviously, there are certain situations that call for quite different interventions.

A major concern is the presence of a major affective illness in one of the partners. One reason for my concern stems from the fact that in one in five couples referred to me, one of the partners, female/male in a 6:1 ratio, has a major depressive episode. Another cause for concern is that the diagnosis is often difficult because the depressive symptomatology has become interwoven with preexisting and now much exacerbated marital pathology. I wonder how many people currently in conjoint therapy across Canada are suffering from undiagnosed major depression?

If I suspect a major affective illness at any time during therapy, I do a diagnostic interview. Once I have made the diagnosis of a major depressive episode, I explain that conjoint therapy is not possible until the depressive episode is treated psychopharmacologically.

In my experience psychotherapy is not effective for a biological depression, and to continue is to have the affected partner at a distinct disadvantage and the marriage at risk.

I undertake to treat the patient individually in brief depression-management visits once every one to two weeks until the person is euthymic, with the understanding that we will resume conjoint therapy after two to three weeks of normal mood. Only when the mood is euthymic can the marital pathology be properly assessed. At the time the diagnosis of depression is made, I have a frank discussion with the couple, giving my diagnosis and treatment recommendations and then discussing the difficulties when one of the dyad becomes an "identified" patient. Although this can present a problem with varying degrees of patient resistance when the diagnosis is initially made, it works well and I have done very effective conjoint therapy following the psychopharmacologic intervention.

In conclusion, I have attempted to describe for you the initial interview in conjoint therapy as I practice it. What I am not able to convey is the richness of the experience, the subtleties, the nuances, the misery, and the humor, so I leave it to you who have been privileged to practice this therapy to fill that in from the well of your own experience.

REFERENCES

1. Framo, J. L. (1982). *Explorations in marital and family therapy.* New York: Springer.
2. Miles, J. E. (1980). Motivation in conjoint therapy. *Journal of Sex and Marital Therapy, 6*(3), 205–213.
3. Broderick, C. B. (1983). *The therapeutic triangle.* Beverly Hills, CA: Sage.

4. Segraves, R. T. (1978). Conjoint marital therapy: A cognitive behavioral model. *Archives of General Psychiatry, 35,* 450–455.

DISCUSSION

Dermott Hurley, M.S.W. *(Victoria Hospital, London)*

I think you will agree that Dr. Miles gave all the richness of his work, and I certainly could feel how he would be with couples when he is dealing with them. I'd like to start with a recent trip to Ireland. I had the opportunity to watch an interview behind a one-way screen (there aren't too many of them in Ireland). I was watching a marital therapist at work. This therapist was having a very awkward time with his client, a woman whom he had worked with in marital therapy for eight years. In the interview, he was saying something like, "Maggie, you can't clam-up on me now, you have a large audience—you've never been hesitant before." She said, "I was hoping for something a little more private," looking at the one-way mirror. It transpired in the discussion about this case later on that the therapist had never seen the husband. He felt that he was doing a very successful job of marital counseling. So there you have it, it is quite simple in terms of values that you take a position!

I wish Dr. Miles could have told us a little bit more about what happens in the initial stages. What he has done is to deepen our own understanding of the crucial beginning stage of therapy and how both sides go about the business of mutual appraisal in deciding about working together. In a very straightforward and lucid way, Dr. Miles tells us about how he assesses expectations. He outlines for us an impressive list of motivations he encounters in his practice. No doubt he would agree that there are many situations in which motivation is mixed.

One of the things that I thought about was the interplay

between resistance and compliance that is so often a part of the initial session in marital therapy. I thought it would be nice to hear him elaborate a little further on the role of the therapist as regulator of marital intimacy, although I'm sure in 10 sessions you are not going to get yourself too caught up in that role. I know in one case that I am treating the task of extricating myself from the role of regulating intimacy in the marriage is becoming a very difficult job. Maybe we should talk about some of our therapeutic failures occasionally.

Dr. Miles sets the scene right from the beginning by offering us his view of conjoint marital therapy. His orientation has both a cognitive behavioral and psychodynamic flavoring rather than an interactional one. He tells us that couples essentially form collusive or reciprocal psychological systems, sometimes based on complementary defenses, for instance, in the hysterical–obsessional marriage. He refers to interlocking object relations to which transferences from family of origin predominate and are generalized to include other members of the opposite sex. Couples seem to induce in the other spouse behavior that is consistent with the internal expectation. A reciprocal behavioral system is set up that actively and continually confirms both spouses' distortions. One would presume that this problem is dealt with on both a cognitive and behavioral level, and I would be most interested in hearing from Dr. Miles how he goes about asking for change on both of these levels.

From what he said so far, the couple are viewed as two individuals who share an important interactional world. For many therapists, it is the interactional field that is the important place for change. By the end of the initial session Dr. Miles offers a well-rounded picture of who the couple are and how workable they might be. In addition to what he said, I personally find it useful to know something about the level of emotional development of both partners, particularly if they form a kind of child–parent marriage or a relationship reflecting a similar level of maturity, their general capacity to form relationships, and whether this is based on realistic expectations and their ability to show both autonomous and dependent behavior. I am especially interested in knowing about separation/individuation experiences and reactions to loss in the lives of both partners.

On the topic of a major affective illness in one partner, I was curious to ask Dr. Miles whether he looks at how the depression may be reinforced by the nondepressed spouse? That is, to what extent does depression in the one partner mask a depression in the other?

I know there are cases that were mentioned by Dr. Martin where somebody in individual therapy ends up feeling much better and the spouse starts complaining about the same symptoms sometime later. Finally, I would like to ask Dr. Miles to comment on what techniques he uses to deal with resistance as a collusive phenomena. The resistant spouse may, in fact, be the one who works the hardest in subsequent sessions so that the presentation at the beginning is not necessarily a comment on the individual's psychological stance, but rather on the collusive nature of the relationship.

Question: I find expectations one of the most difficult aspects in terms of the initial interview. Sometimes the partners do not seem to have any expectations, at least not that they can put into words. How do you facilitate that—do you have any means of getting them to express what they actually expect from therapy?

Dr. Miles: I do not know how to answer the question, since I have not had a problem getting the partners to express their expectations—obviously they are expressed with varying degrees of sophistication. I have not had a problem in getting people to outline their expectations and they are always quite prepared to discuss them further.

Question: First of all, I would like to thank you for a very open, entertaining presentation. There was one thing that intrigued me. You said at the end of the initial interview that you leave it up to them to make a decision about returning. In my experience that is often when the action begins and I have to leave lots of time for this discussion. I wonder what your experience is, because often I find that 20 or 30 minutes is needed to deal with this issue.

Dr. Miles: I say, "I am willing to continue to see you, but the decision is clearly yours, and what you should do is go home and discuss it. If you decide to accept my offer of treatment, please telephone and make a series of four or five weekly appointments." Often, they will make the decision at the end of the first interview, telling me that they would like to continue, but I would still encourage them to discuss it at home. I think this approach helps to underscore the commitment to therapy. It rarely takes more than two or three minutes to deal with this, and if it is "when the action begins" and takes you 20 to 30 minutes it may be that there has not been sufficient "action" prior to your raising this issue.

Question: I think watching how that decision is made is very important. How that happens in my experience is also a clue to how the partners relate to each other, how they handle problems.

Dr. Miles: I agree. It provides another opportunity to observe how they relate to each other, and also to assess motivation.

Question: Can you give us any demographic information about these couples in terms of their social class and cultural background?

Dr. Miles: The couples are from all social classes, but definitely skewed in the direction of upper-middle class.

Question: What are the average number of sessions you have with a couple?

Dr. Miles: It was 12 when I did this retrospective study, but I did that about 2 years ago. I think it probably is a bit higher now and the range could be anywhere from about 3 to 4 minimum up to about 40 to 45.
Question: What are the intervals?
Dr. Miles: Within the limits of everybody's schedule, I try to do one session a week. This is not only administratively convenient, but is in my experience a therapeutically optimum interval.
Question: You seem to have a very active style in the first interview and I find myself wondering if this has evolved—if you have ever at anytime during your experience used a more laid-back style, having couples tell their own story more than imposing the structure? I was not clear how you would deal with a couple who wanted to come back but were both quite ambivalent about the future of the marriage—whether you would alter the assessment procedure or if you would consider seeing them alone, or whether you would alter conjoint therapy with couples where there is considerable ambivalence?
Dr. Miles: In response to your first question, the style of my initial interview has evolved over the past 15 years. I find that having a clear format in mind yields much more useful information, with no sacrifice of the opportunity to observe transactional phenomena. In response to your second question regarding a couple who are ambivalent about the future of their marriage, I would use exactly the same approach. Their ambivalence is much more likely to be made explicit when one is using a structured approach where special questions have been asked about expectations with thoughts regarding separation and motivation. There would be no reason to see them alone; the only difference during therapy would be a focus on, and attempt to resolve, their ambivalence.
Question: I have two questions. The first has to do with

your statement that you will not see either of them individually, with the exception of one spouse who might have an affective disorder. So when you tell them this and add that you will not accept phone calls, I am interested in knowing if you get questions or nonverbal behavior suggesting they have negative feelings about your policy.

Second, when you take the individual histories in the presence of the partner in your second and third visit, what do you do if you come upon an area that seems as if it is a secret?

Dr. Miles: In answer to your first question, of course I have partners who want to be seen alone. The reason for this is often the very reason why these persons are in marital conflict. They cannot talk to each other. They are so afraid of getting in a conflict with the partner that they want to tell me individually about something. Part of the advantage of having a plan is that you are in charge. The plan reinforces for the patients, "Don't worry, I've got a plan and I know what I'm doing." This is very comforting because these people are understandably very apprehensive.

In answer to your second question, I have not had the experience of coming upon "an area that seems as if it is a secret." On those rare occasions when I have seen one spouse alone and become privy to a "secret," which is an item of information that is unknown to the other spouse and would be distressing, I feel my effectiveness as a therapist is severely diminished. I am supposed to be a model of clear communication and straightforward, direct, open, and honest behavior. There is no way that I can sit with a couple when I share a secret with one partner. Furthermore, I do not need to know the "secret." If, for example, one of the spouses is currently involved in an extramarital affair the poor motivation of that partner becomes very obvious by the third or fourth session, and focusing on the motivation usually results in either disclosure or the poor motivation being made absolutely explicit.

Dr. Waring: When you are talking about interviewing, you are obviously talking about being fairly active in an assessment interview. Will you stop a negative interaction between a couple when you ask your question, "How is this fellow a pain in the ass?" If they get into an argument, do you stop that happening in the assessment?

Dr. Miles: Arguments of any consequence rarely break out in the initial interview. Each couple knows they are going to have their turn, and I think the structure helps to reduce the incidence of prolonged negative interaction.

Dr. Waring: It is our experience in training people who are doing their first or second marital assessment, mainly with medical students and others, that unless you help them to stop those kinds of interactions, a negative experience results for the couple. They may not come back, regardless of what happens with the rest of the interview.

Dr. Miles: Yes. What might be said is something like this, "I see what you're doing and you can do that at home, you don't need to be here to do that." Permitting couples to argue longer than necessary to get a sample of that behavior is very counterproductive to effective assessment and therapy.

Question: I was wondering if you could elaborate a little bit more on affairs and how they are revealed. You indicated in a previous response that they come out by the third or fourth session.

Dr. Miles: In my experience, extramarital affairs are most often just one of the many symptoms of a dysfunctional marriage. One should also draw a distinction between a previous affair and a current affair. There may be no need for disclosure of a previous affair. If there is a current affair, it is usually reflected in the individual's motivation and is quite apparent by the fourth or fifth session.

Question: My own experience has been that those couples are sometimes quite willing to expiate guilt by "going along" with marital therapy.

Dr. Miles: Your question clearly relates to what I said about the importance of recognizing "alternative motivations" in my presentation.

Question: The second question I have has to do with the comments you made about intimacy in describing your theoretical framework. I am interested in your experience that in the course of 12 sessions, you feel you are accomplishing change in the capacity to be more intimate. I guess my own impression is that it seems to take longer.

Dr. Miles: Well, sometimes it does. It depends on how quickly the therapist has been able to identify and dissipate the couple's hostile-destructive collusive transactions. When the anger has gone, one is left with two people both wary of intimacy. If they are well motivated, significant improvement in their capacity for intimacy can be achieved relatively quickly in my experience.

Question: I have a comment and then a question. In your initial interview, it seems to me that the line between interviewing and therapy is a fine one. There is a lot of therapy taking place in the first interview, which is perhaps one of the things that makes it effective. As you say, by the end of the interview you have a pretty good intuitive feeling as to whether these people are suitable. I was a little uneasy, however, when you started talking about depression. It seems to me very hard to call that a primary affective disorder when it might be related to events in the therapy. In my experience, sometimes it is a reaction to improvement in the other partner. I would be a little uncomfortable with stopping at that point and labeling one spouse as suffering a major affective problem, and using drugs at that point.

Dr. Miles: I do this if symptoms meet the diagnostic criteria for a major depressive episode.

Question: Do you attempt to relate it to events in the therapy?

Dr. Miles: No, because it is not always clear. The thing that worries me the most is how difficult it is to make the diagnosis. The depressive symptoms become interwoven with the preexisting marital pathology. Often the depressed spouse attributes the symptoms to the partner and is reluctant to accept that the symptoms may or may not be related to the marital pathology. When the affected spouse is euthymic, occasionally there is no longer any marital problem whatsoever. More commonly, the preexisting marital pathology emerges and conjoint therapy can proceed.

Question: Do you find that after the initial interview you are perceived by one member of the couple as being in that person's favor against the other partner, as taking sides?

Dr. Miles: The establishment of a symmetrical relationship is fundamental to effective therapy. If I sense that one partner feels in any way scapegoated, I make it explicit and discuss the issue.

Chapter 4

ASSESSMENT OF MOTIVATION FOR MARITAL THERAPY

Michael Rosenbluth

In individual psychotherapy the issue of motivation for treatment has been a controversial one. While it has been emphasized by Sifneos and others as being of cardinal importance, it has also been suggested that it is a vague concept laden with value judgments and that rather than being useful it has been a means of dismissing patients.[1-3] It has even been suggested that it is of no importance as the therapist has the total responsibility for treatment.[4]

In marital therapy, I will suggest that the assessment of motivation is the central issue both initially and throughout treatment. The particular nature of the dyadic unit having separate and sometimes conflicting conscious and unconscious needs and fears, results in a therapeutic situation where the importance of motivation as a determining factor is paramount. In fact, I will suggest that a main determinant of successful treatment is the therapist being aware of issues regarding motivation for marital therapy. Careful and detailed analysis of the different variables serves to place the therapeutic endeavour on a sure and solid foundation. Insufficient attention to conscious and unconscious factors regarding motivation will result in less successful marital therapy treatment.

Before elaborating, it is necessary to have a clear understanding of what is meant by motivation. I will define motivation and contrast it with different terms to clarify and operationalize the definition. The *Random House College Dictionary*[5] defines a motive in several ways: (1) as something that prompts a person to act in a certain way or that determines volition, (2) as the goal or object of one's actions, (3) as something prompting one to action. The Latin origin of the term is "motivus" which means "serving to move." The dictionary reminds us that there is a difference between a motive, an inducement, and an incentive.[5] While all three terms apply to whatever moves a person to action, they have different connotations. A *motive* is applied mainly to an inner urge that moves or prompts a person to action, while an *inducement* is never applied to an inner urge but is used mainly to discuss opportunities offered by another person or situation, and an *incentive* refers to that which inspires a person in the sense of something offered as a reward.

Reflecting on these dictionary definitions of motives and associated terms, it is interesting to consider that marriage potentially offers all three—positive motives, inducements, and incentives. However, the couple that presents for treatment is not able to actualize the potential inherent in marriage because of the presence of conflict. The work of marital therapy depends on understanding, defining, and sometimes resolving the intrapsychic and interpersonal sources of conflict that make up much of what blocks the utilization of the natural inducements and incentives in marriage. Understanding and clarifying conscious and unconscious variables leads to the improvement of motivation for marital treatment. While initially the conscious motivational factors may emerge more readily and be more important with regard to the seeking of treatment, the unconscious factors related to issues such as intimacy, sex, aggression, and identity may be crucial determinants of the motivational level during the course of treatment and may affect the couple's willingness and capacity to stay in treatment and change.

Before considering this further, we must differentiate between motivation and resistance. Operationally we may contrast motivation to resistance by saying that in the beginning of the assessment, the lack of willingness to engage in marital therapy is seen as a lack of motivation. The work of the assessment is to clarify the factors that contribute to the lack of motivation, and foster an improvement in the level of motivation so that marital therapy can be conducted. At the end of the assessment, while the relevant factors may or may not be elucidated, what remains is whether or not the couple is willing to commit themselves to working on the marriage. After the couple have had an assessment process, which has consisted of the elaboration of motivating factors and blocks, and if at the end of this process the couple is not able to truly make a commitment to marital therapy, operationally this couple may be defined as having a resistance to marital therapy and other treatment options may be considered. Thus, the distinction between a lack of motivation and resistance to treatment is of importance empirically in determining the different treatment options.

What will be considered in this paper is the importance of the therapist paying specific and close attention to the different issues related to motivation and how they influence marital therapy. The paper will be divided into four parts. The first will be the presentation of common motivational constellations. The second will be an outline of some factors affecting motivation. The third will be a discussion of some aspects that influence motivation during the assessment process. The final section will consider the importance of monitoring and improving motivation during the course of treatment.

SPECIFIC MOTIVATIONS FOR MARITAL THERAPY

It is important to consider why the couple seeks treatment. In particular, it is necessary to differentiate the latent from the manifest reason for presentation. In previous articles, Cameron and myself, Smith and Grunebaum, and Miles have described different motivational constellations.[6-8]

1. *Looking for a caretaker.* This describes the situation where the manifest reason for seeking help is marital distress. The latent reason is to have the therapist look after the spouse who has become a burden.

2. *Expiating guilt.* In this situation one spouse is not at all interested in marital therapy but because of guilt feelings about deciding to leave the marriage or due to guilt over a current affair, comes for marital treatment in order to expiate these feelings of guilt. Here coming to treatment is seen as being the least the spouse can do and usually that's true, it *is* the least.

3. *Looking for an ally.* A partner seeks help in standing up to the mate, feeling inadequate to do so.

4. *Looking for reentry.* Here one partner is looking to be declared "sick" or "neurotic" as a means enabling this person to get back into the marriage.

5. *Response to an ultimatum.* In this "or else" situation,

an ultimatum has been issued to the other and seeking treatment is more a wish to respond to the ultimatum than to seek help.

6. *Avoidance of self-observation.* Sometimes seeking marital therapy can be an avoidance of seeking individual therapy which may be indicated but is perceived as being too threatening.

7. *Blaming the spouse.* Here treatment becomes just another opportunity to vent anger and hostility.

8. *Being declared innocent.* Marital therapy is sought to have one partner identified as guilty and the other as innocent.

9. *Marital therapy as a career.* Therapy is seen as a necessary on-going adjunct to marital life.

Thus there are numerous reasons, both conscious and unconscious, that may serve as obstacles to treatment and that must be ferreted out as soon as possible. An understanding of adaptive and maladaptive expectations of treatment is crucial in determining what treatment approach is necessary and what issues will be focused on. Clarifying this initially permits more suitable therapeutic contracts to be established on the basis of more appropriate motivations.

FACTORS AFFECTING MOTIVATION

Different factors affect motivation. Overviewing external and internal issues at the outset of treatment facilitates therapeutic engagement. The factors to be considered are the perception of marital distress, issues related to sex and anger, the presence of malignant factors in the marriage, and developmental and economic considerations.

Marital Distress

The recognition of marital distress, a feeling of personal helplessness to resolve matters, and the belief in the therapist as a possible helper are important constituents of motivation for treatment.[9] Factors affecting these variables include the chronicity of the problem, character structure of the spouses, and cultural values regarding the seeking of help. Thus, the more chronic the problem the less likely the couple is to seek help unless there has been a major recent crisis. Chronicity diminishes the sense that any other state is possible. Related to this is the character structure of the partner, for example, those masochistically inclined may endure the situation because unconscious needs are being gratified. A combination of chronicity and characterologic factors may result in individuals developing a stance of resignation and detachment that precludes their active involvement in psychotherapy.

With regard to the recognition of the need for help, some individuals, because of previous negative developmental experiences, are not capable of believing that their expression of emotional distress will be met by concerned involvement by the therapist. This negative transference may interfere with the seeking of help. In others, cultural factors make turning to the therapist less acceptable. However, if the subjective distress is great and there is a recognition of the need for help, cultural bias can be overcome. Thus for a couple to seek treatment, they must recognize a state of distress, feel helpless to resolve it themselves, and must recognize the therapist as a potential helpgiver.

Sex

The sexual life of the couple must always be assessed in detail not only because there may be sexual problems present but also because operationally the presence of sexual problems can be a critical variant in the level of motivation of the couple. Sexual problems are related to motivation in several ways: First, if there are sexual problems present, the sex drive of one or both partners may cause them to seek treatment when they may not otherwise do so. Many spouses who resign themselves to marital problems increase their motivation if they think that their sexual life will be improved. Second, conscious or unconscious fears of sex may be a factor decreasing the level of motivation to work on sexual or marital problems. This is the converse of the previous situation and tends to occur more often in women. Third, sexual problems may be causing the marital problem and in this way may be a factor necessitating marital intervention. In addition, for some marriage partners, their sexual life together serves a restitutive function within the marriage and when it is lost this causes the couple to seek help so that this aspect of the marriage can be restored. Fourth, there is a great sexual vulnerability that affects individuals. In particular, men who might not otherwise seek marital therapy may become extremely motivated to do so if they are experiencing a sexual problem because it shakes the core of their personality, making them feel extremely vulnerable and inadequate. In this instance, the need for treatment is perceived as urgent. Thus the presence of a sexual problem or conscious or unconscious sexual fears can be crucial determinants in either impeding or promoting the couple's interest in marital therapy.

Anger

The amount and means of dealing with anger in marriage must be assessed. There are many causes for anger in marriage at both the conscious and unconscious level. The opportunities for disappointment, misunderstanding, and rage are considerable. These may be related to more superficial and conscious disappointment but may also relate to unconscious conflict as manifested in projective identifications, blurred ego boundaries and, in the most general sense, transference reactions to the spouse. The feelings provoked may be quite intense. For the purposes of our discussion, the amount of anger present and how it is dealt with is of importance in how it affects the partners' motivational levels. Too high levels of expressed anger on a chronic basis can be corrosive in marital treatment in that it may decrease the motivation for marital therapy of one or both spouses. In this case too little impulse control can erode the formation of a therapeutic alliance. Alternatively, the inability of the spouses to express anger may result in their using withdrawal and resignation as a means of dealing with disappointment and frustration in marriage. Withdrawal and resignation can impair motivational levels, and can cause couples to either not present for treatment or to feel too hopeless about accomplishing anything, and thus terminate treatment prematurely. The conscious recognition, management, and expression of anger must be assessed and dealt with before deficiencies in this area impair the formation of a treatment alliance. Understanding the sources of anger and disappointment, and facilitating improved means of dealing with these feelings can permit marital therapy to proceed.

The Presence of a Malignant Force in Marriage

During the assessment phase it is very important to ascertain whether or not there is what may be termed a malignant force present in the marriage. This includes the presence of an excessive interest outside the marriage or the presence of psychiatric disease. Examples of the former include a spouse having an affair or having already decided to definitely leave the marriage; another example is when the spouse's occupation becomes a subject of inordinate preoccupation. A potentially malignant force in the marriage is the presence of a formally diagnosed psychiatric disease. It is important to determine whether there is a major mental illness present in one or both partners and whether it is being treated appropriately. Undiagnosed psychopharmacologically responsive depressive illness is a good example of a force that when left untreated, can be a malignant force in the marriage and yet when treated can make a very great difference in the marital therapy or even the need for marital therapy.

Other Factors

Other factors regarding motivation relate to the spouse's life cycle, developmental issues, and the reality of economics and alternatives. Considerations regarding life cycle may affect the motivation for marital therapy in numerous ways. While life cycle considerations affect the capacity for involvement and intimacy and therefore affect motivation, what will be mentioned here are situations that need to be noted in terms of the more general effect on the motivation of the couple. Thus, young couples may have trouble committing themselves to the marriage and marital therapy because they have not separated from their families of origin. Older couples with children may seek treatment to resolve difficulties for the sake of the children. Previously married individuals may work harder to stay together because they have already experienced divorce and are determined not to do so again. Professional or work-related goals may have a greater priority at certain times in the partner's life cycle and may diminish motivation to work on relationship concerns. Later on, with these goals consolidated, more attention can be paid to the marriage.

Developmental considerations include the capacity to

live an autonomous life. Individuals who have not fully separated and who fear consciously or unconsciously being alone and the primitive feelings they may associate with this state, may feel obliged to continue in a relationship longer than they might otherwise choose to. While such a situation does not provide a positive motivation for marriage or marital therapy, it does provide an opportunity for growth and change to occur. Conversely, some marriages suffer when an individual, through personal therapy or other circumstances, becomes sufficiently individuated to leave the marriage.

Economic factors need to be considered. The willingness to pay the therapist's fee can be a good indicator of motivation initially and throughout the treatment. Financial considerations also compel couples to live together as they simply cannot afford to separate.

Consideration of the financial possibilities regarding separation is only one aspect of considering the alternatives that the spouses each entertain. Detailed questioning regarding what would happen if separation or divorce occurred can be quite sobering to each spouse or alternately may be quite sobering for the therapist. The need to help couples can at times lead to a blinding countertransference on the part of the therapist. Some couples may find separation or divorce quite attractive, and a careful analysis of this consideration may help both the couple and the therapist be more in tune with the reality of the situation.

VARIABLES IN THE ASSESSMENT AFFECTING MOTIVATION

The assessment phase presents the therapist the opportunity to assess the couple's motivation, while considering the issues described previously. In addition, the therapist may improve motivation by:

1. Clarifying countertransference problems that impede

motivation by collusion with negative motivational constellations.
2. Issue communication challenges to the couple as a means of clarifying and improving motivation.
3. Defining responsibility for the treatment as a means of clarifying and improving motivation.
4. Defining concrete and mutual goals.
5. Setting up a therapeutic interaction that encourages the couple by satisfying immediate needs for nurturance, thus raising motivation and instilling hope.

Countertransference

The therapist's countertransference is an important variable to consider. Therapists must be aware of their conscious and unconscious views of marriage, including their own marriage, those of their parents, and those of their patients. Marital therapy is a very complex process which prompts numerous feelings in the therapist at a conscious and unconscious level and offers numerous occasions for entanglement as there are so many different combinations of transference–countertransference configurations possible.[10] It is necessary not only to overcome the more traditional kind of transference but also to overcome the "futility countertransference." For some psychiatrists, marriage and schizophrenia have the same empirical definition, that is, both are characterized by the four *A*'s—looseness of association, ambivalence, affective disturbance, autism, plus a deteriorating course. Thus one must be fully aware of one's own feelings with regard to marriage in order to be the most effective marital therapist and not have one's countertransference act in collusion with patient's resistance and lower motivation.

Communication

Improved communication improves motivation. In particular, besides the usual work directed at improving communication, I offer the couple what I term a *communication challenge*. I invite them to change their communication in a simple but definite manner. The method is to invite the couple to start talking about their own feelings and their own perceptions rather than their conclusions about their partner's feelings and perceptions. Instead of a provocative mode of communication, for example, "You hate me, you undermine me," I suggest to couples they use a personal mode, for example, "When you do this it makes me feel this," etc. The purpose of this communication challenge is twofold. On the one hand it provides the couple with a more effective means of communicating which is less provocative and antagonistic and allows issues to be clarified rather than battles fought. However, it is also a test of motivation in that it tests the willingness of couples to try something new and listen to the therapist. Couples coming for marital treatment often present at a point where there is little good will shown on either side and this communication challenge serves as a signal from one spouse to the other and from both to the therapist that there is a willingness to try something new to break the negative cycle. Some couples who are so discouraged when they come for treatment can be very encouraged by one spouse being willing to change the communication and take responsibility for doing so.

Responsibility

The capacity of the individuals presenting for marital therapy to be open and honest and willing to look at their own weaknesses and their own contribution to the state of marital distress is essential. While this capacity can be influenced during the course of the assessment and the course of treatment, some degree of self-reflection and assumption of responsibility for problems is essential for marital treatment to proceed. The presence of this kind of responsibility assumption in the assessment phase can be very important for the other spouse to note. It is often very surprising and encouraging for the other spouse and reinforces the motivational level of all parties concerned. A spouse using the marital intervention as an opportunity to express newly gained insight and responsibility for some of his or her own behavior or to accept an interpretation from the therapist can be a very important signal to the other spouse. Nothing can be as encouraging and helpful as for one spouse to hear the other spouse sing a new song, one that includes recognition of some personal responsibility for marital woes rather than the old refrain, "It's your fault." Self-reflection and responsibility assumption are encouraged and reinforced. The couple is told explicitly that they must change themselves if they are to see change in the partner. It is also stressed from the outset and throughout treatment that the responsibility for treatment is the couple's and not the therapist's. This relates to magical expectations of the therapist that interfere with motivation and that will be discussed in more detail later.

Goals

Motivation is improved by formulating with the couple explicit concrete treatment goals and priorities and communicating to the couple the values and beliefs that the therapist holds about the couple's marriage. I have found it helpful to operationalize a number of concepts and reframe a number of the patients' problems toward a more concrete empirical level. The clarity gained by this is encouraging for couples. Thus concepts such as trust, respect, and caring are operationalized in terms of skills necessary to facilitate these feelings. This is important because of the initial state of the couple at the time of presentation. Often they have too much difficulty believing that change can occur with respect to large attitudinal shifts. Breaking these components down to basic skills and work directed at remedying skills deficits rather than trying to tackle huge fundamental problems is more positive, encouraging, and work-promoting, particularly for the demoralized couple.

It is important to work with the couple in determining what the perceived problems are and what reasonable and realistic goals and expectations of each other might be. These goals must be as explicit as possible. While a clear attempt is made to operationalize the goals and make them as concrete as possible, attention is also placed on what is occurring psychodynamically between the members of the couple. Issues regarding conflicts about intimacy, identity, cooperation, the handling of anger, needs for dependency, and autonomy are examined closely. As much as possible these issues are handled on an operational level, seeking to look at communication manifestations as well as tracing the psychodynamic, developmental, and current aspects of these conflicts. During the process of formulating clear goals and priorities and discussing values and beliefs regarding their marriage, it is important to assess how congruent the couple's and the therapist's views of the marital situation and the goals of treatment are. If there is truly a very divergent opinion at the outset, either between the spouses themselves or between the couple and the therapist, it remains to be seen how much can be accomplished.

Nurture and Hope

By the time a couple comes for treatment both individuals usually are feeling very psychologically battered, and are often full of bitterness, anger, disappointment, hopelessness, and rage. The developmental antecedents of these affects need to be understood so they can be handled better and be less corrosive to the marriage. Communication work must be done to decrease the expressed hostility and provocativeness. It is also necessary for the couple to have someone to relate to and be a nurturing source until they are both in a better position to do this for each other.

This job falls to the therapist, who must be prepared to assume it. In general, understanding the couple's problems from a mutual perspective, giving some perspective through exploring and interpreting the origins of the problems, being fair and impartial to both sides, being reassuring, and expressing hope are all in the service of nurturing the couple.

It can be suggested that both individuals have an intense hunger for a self-object to help them feel whole and to console them and soothe them. The pain and disappointment of marital distress is interfering with these normal mechanisms. Thus one role of the therapist, who does not have a backlog of anger or disappointment toward the couple, is to be a self-object for both individuals in the marriage. This function provides a soothing and nurturing which decreases the psychological isolation of each individual and can increase the motivation to facilitate the spouses working on the problem more constructively and working toward taking over the self-object function for each other. The work of treatment is to help the couple disengage from their projective identifications and blurred symbiotic boundaries. The therapist encourages the couple to communicate differently and relate in a more differentiated way to each other, and to work through change or accept deficits. The couple become more able to be self-objects for each other while strengthening and preserving their own respective selves.

Thus the assessment phase is not a static one. The process begun by the therapist and the couple venting and exploring intense feelings, reframing problems, clarifying responsibility, setting goals, working on current communication, and the beginning of a healing process serves to indicate that a new momentum is being developed to reverse the negative spiral that has led to the seeking of marital therapy. The reassurance that there is a therapist willing to nurture, listen, arbitrate, help, and educate can be very encouraging to the demoralized couple. As Jerome Frank has pointed out, the instillment of hope is one of the fundamental processes in psychotherapy.[11] This is certainly true in marital therapy.

AFTER THE ASSESSMENT

The assessment of motivational factors is not limited only to the assessment phase of treatment. There is a continuous need to monitor the level of motivation because it is usually an accurate barometer of psychodynamic issues that are developing and need to be addressed. During the course of treatment, motivation should be maintained or increased, as it is heightened by progress and the increasing curiosity the couple experiences about themselves during the therapeutic process. The barometer function of motivation refers to resistances developing in the course of treatment that decrease the motivational level. The determination of the sources of resistance, usually basic conflictual issues, comprises an important part of the work of treatment.

In addition, during the course of therapy, there are different levels of motivation that occur and one of the functions of treatment is to shift the level of motivation from the more primitive to the more mature level. The capacity to engage in a psychotherapeutic process lies along a spectrum—from the couple's magical expectation that the therapist will solve all their problems, to a wish to have the therapist act as a powerful parental figure, to a desire to work together cooperatively to determine what is happening and what is to be done. During the course of treatment, specific attention to this parameter, as manifested in the spouses' relationship to and expectation of the therapist, offers an opportunity to lay a more solid foundation for marital therapy. The couple's magical or parental cravings can be examined and through interpretation the level of expectation can be shifted to a more mature orientation. The more mature the level of expectation, the more ambitious the therapist and couple can be toward accomplishing change. The less mature the motivation and the greater the craving for magic, the more limited will be the goals.[6,12]

CONCLUSION

The assessment of motivation in marital therapy is the central issue at the beginning and throughout the course of marital therapy. I have presented a survey of different motivational constellations that have to be listened for and attended to. I have reviewed how considering variables related to conflict areas such as sex and aggression, and factors regarding the life cycle, and the perception of alternatives affect motivation for treatment. Consideration has also been given to interactive variables, with regard to the therapist's countertransference, communication, the clarification of goals and responsibility, and issues relating to nurturing the couple and restoring hope which can thereby improve motivation.

I have suggested that establishing what conscious and unconscious factors motivate a couple to seek treatment, and improving and monitoring that motivation, is an important ongoing issue in marital therapy, serves as a barometer of progress, and indicates when new conflictual areas are emerging.

The clarification of the different variables that affect motivation can be seen as the central process of the work of marital therapy. If the motivation is there and is being facilitated by the therapist then the work of the couple in treatment proceeds. If the motivation is not there, neither is the couple. While psychoanalysis has been likened to a long voyage, marital therapy may be seen as a short trip but one where all systems must be "go" in order to facilitate getting to the destination. The assessment of motivation may then be seen as the checking of whether all systems are indeed in a state of readiness before embarking, and indeed throughout the course of the trip.

REFERENCES

1. Sifneos, P. (1978). Motivation for change. A prognostic guide for successful psychotherapy. *Psychotherapy and Psychosomatics, 29,* 293–298.
2. Silverman, S. (1964). The role of motivation in psychotherapeutic treatment. *American Journal of Psychotherapy, 18,* 212–229.
3. Holt, W. (1967). The concept of motivation for treatment. *American Journal of Psychiatry, 123,* 1388–1394.
4. Kaiser, H. (1955). The problem of responsibility in psychotherapy. *Psychiatry, 18,* 205–211.
5. *Random House College Dictionary* (Rev. Ed.) (1980). New York: Random House.
6. Rosenbluth, M., Cameron, P. (1981). Assessment, commitment and motivation in marital therapy. *Canadian Journal of Psychiatry, 26,* 151–154.
7. Smith, J. W., & Grunebaum, H. (1976). The therapeutic alliance in marital therapy. In H. Grunebaum & J. Christ (Eds.), *Contemporary marriage: Structure, dynamics and therapy.* Boston: Little, Brown.
8. Miles, J. (1980). Motivation in conjoint therapy. *Journal of Sex and Marital Therapy, 6,* 205–213.
9. Stunkard, A. (1961). Motivation for treatment: Antecedents of the therapeutic process in different cultural settings. *Comparative Psychiatry, 2,* 140–147.
10. Guttman, H. (1982). Transference and countertransference in conjoint couple therapy: Therapeutic and theoretical implications. *Canadian Journal of Psychiatry, 27,* 92–97.
11. Frank, J. (1973). *Persuasion and healing. A comparative study of psychotherapy.* Baltimore: The Johns Hopkins University Press.
12. Rado, S. (1965). The relationship of short-term psychotherapy to developmental stages of motivation and stages of treatment behav-

ior. In L. Wolberg (Ed.), *Short-term psychotherapy*, New York: Grune & Stratton.
13. Wolberg, L. R. (1967). *The technique of psychotherapy* (2nd Ed.). New York: Grune and Stratton.

DISCUSSION

Reid Finlayson, M.C.
(University of Western Ontario)

First, I want to say how much I enjoyed the paper. I had an opportunity to read it and also to hear it. A lot of thought went into the paper and I appreciate that very much.

It seems to me that the paper was a discussion of marital therapy from an intrapsychic and from an interpersonal viewpoint. I was concerned at first because I detected in the tone of the paper very little reference to the sort of general systems theory idea of family and marital therapy, which I have been fairly familiar with—the work of people like Ackerman, Bowen, Minuchin, Haley, and many others. The difficulty is that motivation is not considered very much in that literature. I think the general systems theorists hold that there is some sort of crisis that is responsible for the couple coming to therapy. Once the couple has arrived for therapy, the tendency is for them to resist any change in their current functioning, and the function of the therapist is to try to facilitate some change to a more adaptive or healthier level of functioning. I think in general systems theory that the task of the therapist is to create a crisis that helps to facilitate change.

I wanted to make a comment about the various motivational configurations that lead the couple to come for help. The four factors in these categories seem to reflect two issues. One, the concern about a crisis situation that led the couple to come for help at this particular time, that has to be considered, and then try to look at what is the basic underlying problem. Dr. Waring has done some very worthwhile work in tracing the importance of intimacy and lack of it in human relations, particularly in marriage. I would suggest that deficiencies in intimacy may be a common denominator to the motivational factors that are described.

I personally have a little bit of confusion around the use of transference and countertransference in interpersonal or systems terms. I'm on a little steadier ground when those terms are used to describe feelings and interactions between a therapist and a patient on a one-to-one basis. There is no question though that the ideas of countertransference and transference occurring toward individuals and toward the couple themselves do occur. I do think that Bowen in the family therapy literature has described these relationships well in terms of issues of triangularization between the members of the couple and between the couple and the therapist. I wanted to mention too that Claghorn and Levine from McMaster University quite some time ago discussed the training requirements for family therapists. I think those training requirements involve a need to be familiar with individual psychodynamics as well as interpersonal or family therapy theory.

The next thing I wanted to comment on was that I think there is a need for more research in the area of marital therapy. I think it would be very interesting to evaluate motivation of a couple presenting for marital therapy and then to follow through and see what the actual outcome is and how that relates to the initial motivation. Perhaps this could be done by a questionnaire or some other means. In the individual therapy field it is kind of paralleled, in my mind at least, by the work that Dr. Lazare did at the Massachusetts General Hospital with individuals walking into the outpatient clinic and presenting complaints. He was able to come up with a list of categories of what motivated people to come for treatment and it wasn't the complaints that they initially presented with, as you all know. Lazare's idea was to first gain the person's confidence and establish some sort of rapport and then somehow ask the question, "Look, what are you really here for, what can I possibly do to help?" Then the next part of the assessment or beginning treatment involves actually negotiating what people need or think they need, lined up with what the therapist can offer. There may be something parallel to that research that could be attempted in the marital therapy area. At least I think it is a very interesting parallel.

I want to mention in the motivating factors that I think it is very important to ascertain whether there is an abuse of alcohol or other drugs on the part of one or other of the partners. I don't think that was directly alluded to. In my understanding of Dr. Rosenbluth's ideas, perhaps the use of alcohol and drugs could be discussed under the anger category and the difficulty in handling anger. I think that is a sufficiently common problem in my experience that the issue of using drugs or alcohol comes up as a determinant of motivation in on-going treatment at times.

In conclusion, I would just like to reiterate that I think the ideas that Dr. Rosenbluth has presented are very interesting. I think the paper leans on psychodynamic ideas with a lot of reference to interpersonal concepts. I would agree that an effective marital therapist requires a solid base of training in individual assessment and therapy. I also suggest that the ideas should be tested experimentally. I think the future of marital therapy depends on our ability to demonstrate the utility of our theoretical formulations.

Question: I would like to know if Michael, or anybody else here, is familiar with any attempts at quantifying, by means of questionnaires, motivation at the beginning of marital therapy and correlating that with outcome? Has anybody tried that? Is anyone familiar with that?

Dr. Rosenbluth: There has been little work done in in-

Assessment of Motivation for Marital Therapy 77

vestigating the issue of motivation for marital therapy from a formal research perspective. Partly this relates to general difficulties doing marital therapy research, but also reflects difficulties with the conscious and unconscious variables reflected in the motivational level. Certainly I would agree with the call for more research into this area.

Question: Dr. Rosenbluth, with respect to your motivational constellations I wonder whether any of them in themselves constitute contraindications for marital therapy—for example, whether therapists sometimes might say that they don't want to collude with the couple's looking for a caretaker?

Dr. Rosenbluth: That is an interesting question because the whole issue of indications and contraindications that you were pointing out this morning is a very complicated question. I think we all have our own concept of how absolute, how rigid we want to be about contraindications. I don't think that there are absolute contraindications in the list that I cited. I think the point of the motivational constellation is to be mindful that the reason that you are in the office seeing the couple may be quite different than the reason the couple is in the office seeing you. If you can start from there and decipher what is going on, then I think there is a lot of room for good work to be done, depending on how flexible the system can be.

Question: In the context of your own clinical practice, if in the initial assessment you determine that perhaps one of the marital partners is really there for the purpose of expiating guilt, how often will that motivation or can that motivation change to another motivation?

Dr. Rosenbluth: I've had more success if that motivation is present if I work on this in individual therapy first to clear the way for marital therapy, rather than vice versa. My own experience has been that if one member of the couple isn't really there then they are both not there. There is very little that I can do at that time in terms of helping them if they really have their heart in their job or they have their heart in other parts of their anatomy in an involvement with someone else. My experience has been that if a proper assessment is done, this may facilitate engagement in treatment at a later date. When things change, people come back and then some more useful work can be done. I think a lot of the time, particularly with residents who are new in marital therapy, they are enthusiastic to save the marriages. They want to have a case for supervision and aren't listening to the fact that they are working far harder than the couple. I always emphasize this with these residents, and I always emphasize up front to the couple that it is their marriage, not mine, and that the two people working the hardest have to be them not me. It is helpful I think to be up front because I think people do have some idea that simply by coming to therapy there is this tremendous power that is going to happen when they walk through the doors of the hospital.

Comment: I just wanted to say that Carl Whitaker, in one of his more famous interventions with a couple where one member is having an affair, said, "Well, at least somebody is doing something about this awful marriage." I think the virtue of Michael's approach is that he is talking about the interactive and constantly fluctuating change of motivation. You're not talking about it as a state or as a trait, you're talking about it as a stage that fluctuates and that is partially determined by the therapist's reactions. Because it isn't just them, it is you and them together forming a new unit, which creates something very different.

Dr. Waring: A question to both Michael and Jim, who talked about the same topic this morning. When you identify one of these patterns, a pattern such as coming

for expiation of guilt, how do you articulate that or *do* you articulate that to the couple, and what happens?
Dr. Rosenbluth: I find it very helpful to share my understanding with the couple in a manner as explicit as possible so that we can work together to change the motivational level. Understanding the motivational constellation permits couples to have an opportunity to shift to a more adaptive level. Recognizing and resolving the issues that diminish motivation is an important part of the treatment process.
Dr. Miles: I really enjoyed the paper. I was certainly relating to the things that Michael identified. I think it is interesting to take a look at Wolberg's book on psychotherapy.[13] The section on motivation is relatively brief and deals primarily with juveniles, psychopaths, and criminals. There is almost an assumption that anyone else that presents for psychotherapy in your office is motivated and shares the same goals as the therapist. I was also happy to hear you say that motivation isn't only an issue in the initial assessment session, but that it is an issue throughout therapy.

Chapter 5

TYPES OF MARITAL THERAPY IN PSYCHIATRIC PRACTICE

Michael F. Myers

I will present three ways of classifying types of marital therapy. Much of this material has been published elsewhere but is presented here to orient the reader and to provide a quick review. None of the classifications is mutually exclusive. There is some overlap from one type to another. Later in the chapter I will describe specifically my approach to couples for assessment and treatment.

TYPOLOGY BASED ON THEORETICAL ORIENTATION

There are three commonly described theoretical approaches to marital therapy: behavioral, systems, and psychoanalytic–psychodynamic.

Behavioral

This approach is based on learning theory principles and includes such concepts as reinforcement and modeling. The therapist creates and maintains a positive therapeutic alliance, negotiates treatment objectives with the couple, helps them agree on limited behavioral goals between visits, and then examines their attempts to achieve them. The main proponents of this approach have been Liberman,[1] Stuart,[2] and Jacobson.[3]

Systems

General systems theory is based on the principle that the whole is an integrated entity and not simply the sum of its parts. In other words, a change in one part brings about a change somewhere else in the system. One member of a couple will be affected by changes in the other spouse, changes in the children, or changes in the environment. The main contributors to this model have been Bowen[4] and Minuchin.[5]

Psychoanalytic–Psychodynamic

This approach addresses intrapsychic factors. Most workers in this area attempt to make some distinction between "psychoanalytic" and "psychodynamic," although in some writings these terms are used interchangeably. Most commonly, the term psychoanalytic refers specifically to Freud in regard to principles of investigation and the particular technique used as a method of treatment. In this respect, psychoanalytic theories and techniques are psychodynamic, but not all psychodynamic theories and techniques are psychoanalytic, for example, those of Sullivan, Klein, and Jung.

The psychoanalytic–psychodynamic perspective states that intrapsychic factors (both consciously and unconsciously) exert a significant effect on object choice in marriage as well as affecting the quality of the relationship and interactions between various members of the family. One of the original workers in this area was Dicks,[6] followed later by Martin,[7] and Sager.[8]

Additional Typology Based on Theoretical Orientation

Often included under systems theory is communications theory, the main proponents being Haley[9] and Satir.[10] Marital problems are seen in terms of transactional communications, often with discrepancies between verbal and nonverbal behavior. Spiegel[11] has analyzed marital interactions with principles of role theory. Equilibrium is maintained by reciprocity of roles. A feminist approach to marital therapy encompasses many principles of social role and sex role theory and argues that traditional marriage values, rules, and expectancies have been unhealthy for women.[12] A feminist approach espouses egalitarian principles and is particularly germane during this contemporary era of rapidly changing roles for men and women both within and outside the boundaries of marriage.

TYPOLOGY BASED ON FORMAT, APPROACH, OR TECHNIQUE

Listed on the next page are several commonly employed approaches to marital therapy.

Types of Marital Therapy

1. *Individual.* In this approach only one member of the couple is in treatment. Any of the above theoretical orientations may be used. However, individual treatment usually refers to those patients who are in either classical psychoanalysis or long-term psychoanalytically oriented psychotherapy.

2. *Consecutive.* This approach is not as common as was once used and refers to each member of the couple being in psychotherapy but one follows the other at the conclusion of the first partner's treatment. Each member of the couple sees the same therapist.

3. *Concurrent.* In this form of marital therapy each member of the couple is in treatment simultaneously with the same therapist.

4. *Collaborative.* In this approach each member of the couple is in treatment with different therapists who are in regular contact with each other, with each partner's consent.

5. *Conjoint.* This is the most commonly used approach to marital therapy. It means that both partners are seen together at the same time by the same therapist.

6. *Combined.* This approach encompasses concurrent and conjoint therapy and is a flexible model with important advantages.

7. *Couples' groups.* This form of marital therapy uses principles of group therapy in treating couples. It is particularly advantageous for couples with chronically maladaptive and egosyntonic patterns of communication.

The above typology also encompasses the use of cotherapy. There are many different types of cotherapy situations. Cotherapists may be of the same sex or the opposite sex. They may be husband and wife. They may be supervisor and supervisee. They may be professional colleagues of the same or different discipline. What is most important, however, is that the nature of the cotherapy relationship is fundamental in its impact on the transference manifestations of the couple in treatment.

TYPOLOGY BASED ON SPECIFICITY OF COUPLES OR GOALS IN TREATMENT

This typology includes any of the already mentioned theoretical orientations or therapeutic approaches; there are common problem areas or themes that cut across other diagnostic schemes. I have listed some of these couple situations but the list is not intended to be exhaustive.

1. Alcoholism in one or both partners.
2. Major psychopathology in one or both partners (example: bipolar affective disorder, borderline personality organization, schizophrenia, Alzheimer's disease, and so forth.
3. Gay male or lesbian couples.
4. Bisexuality in one or both partners.
5. Dual-career couples (coprofessional couples).
6. Sexual dysfunction in one or both partners of a couple.
7. Separation or divorce therapy.
8. Interracial or interfaith couples.
9. Remarriage marital therapy.

AN INTEGRATED MODEL

This is the model with which I am most comfortable and most experienced. Couples coming for marital therapy are so diverse in background, socioeconomic reference group, duration of symptomatology, motivation for treatment, availability of ego resources, and stage of marital cycle that a flexible model is really quite essential. With some couples a simple and straightforward behavioral approach to marital conflict will work beautifully; in other couples the same approach will achieve nothing or will be deemed inappropriate or insulting. A period of conjoint approach for some couples is essential; with other couples the same approach is impossible or damaging. The marital therapist must continually monitor the effectiveness of a particular approach and recognize when it is not working. When switching to another format the therapist must always explain very carefully to each member of the couple the reasons for trying a different method.

My approach to marital therapy is a short-term one, that is, the average couple is seen for a total of approximately six to 10 visits over a three to four months period. Initial interviews are conjoint ones, followed by one individual visit for each partner, and the follow-up visits are generally conjoint as well. When and if indicated, further individual visits are scheduled as therapy progresses.

The Initial Interview

During the first interview I attempt to obtain some idea of the surface complaints that the couple brings to treatment. I am also interested in understanding each partner's sense of the problem areas, and whether they are in agreement on these. It is also important to determine the length of symptomatology and whether the spouses have some thoughts about possible contributing factors to the surface complaints. I learn whether any previous marital therapy has been obtained and what each person's feelings were about that treatment.

If there have been previous separations I like to acquire some information about those separations, what the reasons for separating were, and the circumstances that led to reunion. I try to obtain some sense of the couple's shared interests and also determine what individual and separate interests each member of the couple has. How committed each person is to the marriage is an important consideration as well as each individual's commitment to marital therapy.

If time permits, in the first interview I like to get a little bit of background regarding the relationship. For instance: How did the partners meet? How long was their courtship? Did problems arise during the courtship? Did they live together before marriage? How was that period? Was their early sexual experience together satisfying? Were there any problems? Has there been a change in the sexual pattern, for example, in the frequency and quality of their lovemaking over the course of the marriage? If so, in what ways? Are there any specific sexual dysfunctions in either or both individuals? If so, how does the other partner feel about this? Do they feel that changes in their sexual relationship may be related to other problem areas or external stresses? How was their sexual relationship affected by pregnancy and the postpartum period?

Sometimes during the first conjoint interview it is possible to begin to make an early psychodynamic assessment of their relationship. I try to get some sense of the relative maturity of each partner as well as a beginning sense of their characteristic ego defenses. I am interested in knowing how much projection, denial, rationalization, and so on are used; at this point I begin to assess each partner's ego strength relative to the other.

The Individual Visits

Individual visits equalize the amount of time spent alone with the therapist. Rapport is strengthened and neither partner feels "short-changed" or "one-down." Each partner is given an opportunity to tell his or her story separately without the other partner contradicting or censoring. The therapist is also able to obtain information from each partner that has not been shared with the spouse and may be critical to the assessment, treatment approach, and prognosis. Some examples of such information are undisclosed previous marriages, previous pregnancies and abortions, previous psychiatric treatment, extramarital sexual activity, and homosexuality.

I use individual visits to obtain selective details about the individual's personal and family histories. I like to have some sense of each partner's ability to cope with frustrations, to adapt to stress, and to handle disappointment. I also try to get a sense of each partner's level of self-confidence and self-image. Each partner's relative maturity as well as capacity for empathy are important to determine. What level of separation and individuation has been achieved by each partner and how capable is each partner of independence? What are their respective capacities for love and how able are they to accept support from each other?

With regard to family history, I like to obtain some information regarding each partner's family of origin. What is each patient's perception of his or her parents' marriage or marriages? How happily married are or were the parents? Have there been any separations or divorces in the families of origin? How did the parents resolve their differences? Were there frequent arguments, physical violence, or mutual withdrawal? What were the role assumptions of each parent? Was the father the sole or principal wage earner? Was the mother at home full-time while the patient was growing up? Did she return to paid work later? Was there strict division of labor in the home based on sex? How were the finances controlled? Did the parents spend leisure time together? Is there any family history of alcoholism or psychiatric illness? What are the parents' attitudes toward sex? Was sex discussed openly in the home? Are there any siblings? How are their marriages?

With regard to each partner's personal history I attempt

to determine if there were any developmental problems during childhood. How was the patient's social life during adolescence? When did dating begin? Were there any problems involved in dating? Were there any serious long-term relationships before marriage? How was the patient's first sexual experience? How much sexual experience, if any, did the patient have with others before meeting the marital partner? Were there any problems with this? Have there been any previous marriages? If so, when did the marriages occur and what was the duration of the marriages? Were there children by a previous marriage? What were the reasons for separation and divorce? Was there an adequate time between the divorce and the present relationship for resolution and some autonomy to develop?

It is essential that the therapist not overlook clinical illness in one or both of the partners. This is most likely to occur when tensions are very high in the marriage, separation may be imminent, and both partners are demanding immediate couples intervention. The therapist quickly becomes embroiled in the urgency of the situation and fails to obtain a proper history and make a careful assessment of each individual. Therefore, symptomatic and partly disguised illness in one of the partners may be missed. Some examples of illnesses are: clinical depression, early hypomania, undiagnosed alcoholism, a paranoid disorder, and early dementia. If a primary and individual illness is uncovered then it must be treated first; it is then possible that the marital tensions will decrease or cease. Marital therapy may not be necessary (except for explaining diagnostic and treatment details to the spouse).

Follow-up Visits

Marital therapy is comprised of three different phases: initial, middle, and termination. The number of visits will vary from one couple to the next but most marital therapists tend to employ a once-weekly schedule of visits. My approach to couples is that they are entirely responsible for the forthcoming visit. In other words, I tell them that I expect them to come to the next visit with an agenda or theme or problem area that they wish to work on together. I act as a catalyst to assist them with exploration and understanding of that particular problem issue. I also suggest (and sometimes insist) that they set aside a couple of hours, preferably outside of the home between visits, to discuss the visit that they have just had as well as to prepare for the forthcoming visit. Their ability to go along with this suggestion will vary with their level of resistance, habitual avoidance patterns, degree of motivation, secondary gain, and rapport with the therapist.

I consider my roles and/or responsibilities in marital therapy to include the following: helping to clarify the problems, facilitating solutions, providing perspective, attacking demoralization, giving reassurance, allowing ventilation of pent-up feelings by each partner, promoting self-disclosure, assisting the couple with basic communication skills, encouraging the personal growth and autonomy of each partner, assisting each partner to meet the other's unmet needs, and being aware of and sensitive to gender issues in psychotherapy.

The termination phase begins some time before actual ending of the work. This is discussed openly and visits are scheduled less and less often. As in all psychotherapy, a certain amount of regression is to be expected. I always leave the door open for couples to return together or individually in the future as necessary.

CONCLUSION

In this paper I have attempted to provide only a brief outline of various theoretical and pragmatic approaches to marital therapy. This is the science, the empiricism, the "academic stuff" of learning and practicing marital therapy. What has not been highlighted is the highly abstract and nebulous ingredient, the art of marital therapy—that magic ingredient that is a part of *all* psychotherapies—that essential matrix of innumerable variables which hopefully helps couples most of the time but unfortunately harms couples some of the time.

What are some of these variables? Why do couples rate Doctor X as a savior and Doctor Y as a jerk? How much do issues like where the therapist trained, the particular discipline or mode of training, years of experience, age, marital status, gender, therapist's appearance (thin versus paunchy, latter-day hippie versus three-piece suit, bearded versus no facial hair, pants versus dress), office setting and decor, therapist's personality, therapist's ethnic and racial group, and patient expectancies and motivation matter?

There are no black-and-white answers to these questions. These and many other factors are dynamically important and come into play a little of the time or a lot of the time with particular couples. What is crucial for all of us who work in this field, and is highly instrumental in our effectiveness as therapists, is how we evolve professionally and personally throughout our career years. Our job is to remain flexible, to keep abreast of the literature, to reflect, to examine our own marriages, to ask for assistance, to avoid premature closure, and most emphatically to listen to our patients.

REFERENCES

1. Liberman, R. (1970). Behavioral approaches to family and couple therapy. *American Journal of Orthopsychiatry, 40,* 106–118.
2. Stuart, R.B. (1969). Operant interpersonal treatment for marital discord. *Journal of Consulting and Clinical Psychology, 33,* 675–682.
3. Jacobson, N.S. (1977). Problem-solving and contingency contracting in the treatment of marital discord. *Journal of Consulting and Clinical Psychology, 45,* 92–100.

4. Bowen, M. (1976). Theory in the practice of psychotherapy. In P.J. Guerin (Ed.), *Family therapy: Theory and practice*. New York: Gardner.
5. Minuchin, S. (1974). *Families and family therapy*. Cambridge, MA: Harvard University Press.
6. Dicks, H.V. (1967). *Marital tensions*. New York: Basic Books.
7. Martin, P. (1976). *A marital therapy manual*. New York: Brunner/Mazel.
8. Sager, C. (1976). *Marriage contracts and couple therapy*. New York: Brunner/Mazel.
9. Haley, J. (1977). *Problem solving therapy*. San Francisco: Jossey-Bass.
10. Satir, V. (1964). *Conjoint family therapy*. Palo Alto, CA: Science and Behavior Books.
11. Spiegel, J. (1971). *Transactions: The interplay between individual, family and society*. New York: Science House.
12. Laws, J.L. (1975). A feminist view of marital adjustment. In A.S. Gurman and D.G. Rice (Eds.), *Couples in conflict*. New York: Jason Aronson.

DISCUSSION

Edward M. Waring, M.D.
(University of Western Ontario)

I like your concept that you are doing relationship therapy and that you need some flexibility. This involves a certain complexity: complexity of attitudes, complexity of thought, and complexity of matching client characteristics to therapy and therapist characteristics. There aren't simplistic rights and wrongs about types of therapy. I would emphasize that at various ages and stages of the marriage you may be doing very different interventions with spouses, the couple, or the family.

You introduce some concepts from sociology and social psychology about marriage. Psychiatrists sometimes neglect the contributions being made by academic sociology and psychology.

I would like to add that a lot of the work done with

marriages by many professionals consists of information giving and simple ventilation of one side of the story or both sides of the story. Marital counseling is still the predominant kind of marital therapy offered to most couples who seek help. There are some articles by Dominion in the *British Medical Journal* that offer some straightforward factual information, advice about types of marriages, and advice about how to counsel people with practical problems. There was a series of 12 very short articles in the *British Medical Journal* in 1982 that I recommend.

One aspect of Dr. Myers's paper deserves comment. I see couples conjointly initially. I have absolutely no success whatsoever by then doing individual assessment. Maybe this is a difference of attitudes, style, or personality between you and me. Maybe you do something differently in individual sessions that I neglect to do, or vice versa, or maybe I do something wrong in individual sessions. I find that it is difficult for me to help couples if one spouse has confided a secret I cannot reveal in conjoint sessions. Perhaps this issue merits further debate.

Now coming back to your organization. I'm going to ask some questions. Why have most authors who have written about marital therapy written about types of therapy under the three broad contexts of psychodynamic, behavioral, or systems therapy? All of those theories came from totally different clinical or research bases than the study of relationships. Systems theory came from biology, psychodynamic theory came from the understanding of the unconscious of a specific group of patients, and behavioral therapy came from animal experiments. Viennese neurotics, rats, and biological systems are not couples. Why have there been so few attempts to try and develop theoretical constellations built on heterosexual relationships? I wonder if others believe there is something intrinsically different between couples, rats, and Viennese neurotics? Jung, for example, wrote some fascinating things about marriage. His writings are not part of the theoretical base for marital therapy from a psychoanalytic perspective. Jung was very fatalistic about marriage. He wrote from his personal experience that his mother's depression was caused by her poor marriage to his father, a clergyman. He argues that males can never have a real interpersonal relationship with a woman until they come to grips with their conscious and unconscious *anima*, their feminine side. He argued that no female can have a genuinely mature relationship with a male until they come to grips with their unconscious *animus*. This simple idea has never formed part of the theoretical construct in psychoanalysis. The same observation is true with systems theory and behavior theory. Transposing these ideas from other contexts, nobody has worked very hard at making them relative to couples. So this is a plea for examining these simplistic notions and trying to come to grips with a more complex theory that relates to heterosexual relationships over time.

My final comment you raised yourself, which is the question of therapist effects compared to therapy effects. I'm sure that all of us who have listened today believe these presenters would improve our relationships, regardless of the type of therapy that they are offering. We have all enjoyed listening to some very experienced, bright, humanistic, and charismatic people. However, somewhere in North America there must be one marital therapist who is inhumane, nonempathic, nongenuine, and has no capacity for unconditional positive regard. Unfortunately, that individual has never written about their work! I can't blame this person at all! I believe there is some truth to this parable and there must be a proportion of marital therapists that do not have these personal qualities demonstrated by our speakers. I think we have to ask what type of therapy is going to be effective as practiced by therapists who lack these positive attributes? I'm addressing the issue of type of therapy versus therapist. One never sees a report of an ineffective therapist in a journal. I'm going to break that habit tomorrow by telling you about an ineffective therapy I've been practicing.

Finally, we have heard today that concurrent or combined therapy fell into disfavor. Nobody ever bothered to document why it was ineffective! What could we have learned from its ineffectiveness? I'm really raising three questions that I think you started to raise in your paper. First, the issue of complexity in theories—if we are going to have types of therapies for couples, surely we need types of theories for couples that are more relevant to relationships. Second, we have to look at types of therapies versus different therapists. What type of therapy is going to be effective for me if I am one of these inhumane, inexperienced therapists without too much personal skill? Finally, my experience has been that the most common reason for failure in marital therapy is an ineffective match between couple, therapist, and therapy. Matching the expectations and qualities of the couple to the expectations and qualities of the therapist and matching these to the most effective type of therapy is a problem that remains to be resolved. I enjoyed your talk very much and now will open the discussion period.

Question: Dr. Waring, you've done some work on studying happily married couples, which is perhaps more practical than studying the neurotic Viennese or rats. Could you tell us some of the characteristics of people who are happily married?

Dr. Waring: To put it in a nutshell, those couples had eight characteristics. Their marital relationship is the most important relationship in their life—everything else comes second, including their careers and children. When these people come in for the interview they have a sense of humor, there is an atmosphere of being relaxed. They are compatible; they have similar values, similar interests, and similar backgrounds. They express affection openly, they disclose their private selves to one another, and they can resolve differences of opinion. I think your point is well taken. You have to learn both from the couples that are happily married and from the couples who have problems—you learn lessons from both of these groups.

Question: I'm a bit concerned about your definition of a happy marriage because it encroaches on an area that I find myself getting more interested in. In my practice I have an opportunity to see children and young adolescents with complaints that could be labeled as functional. In my opinion these complaints are related to my patients' attempts to fit into these happy marriages. I think that one thing we may tend to forget in marital therapy is that these people may arrive at a very good marital relationship that works very well for them as a couple, but that has consequences for the children. I think we tend not to stand back and take a look at these marriages from the standpoint of a six, eight, or 10-year-old child. How is that child able to fit into the system that the parents have worked out for their mutual advantage? In regard to your discussion of systems, I was wondering if you ever considered eventually, toward the termination phase, of trying to get the spouses involved in some sort of family therapy. I often ask my patients, both individuals and couples, this question: Twenty years from now when your son or daughter is lying on the analyst's couch, tell me how you think the son or daughter will describe your marriage as it appeared to him or her as a child? This is an attempt to try and get the marriage partners to see the dynamics of their marriage from the standpoint of a child who is trying to fit happily into it. As I see these children with their somatic complaints, I think that this is something that isn't always thought about.

Dr. Myers: There are many different levels to your question. Let me respond to it in two different ways. First, in my practice I'm often struck by the number of couples I see who are so preoccupied with their distress that my attempts to understand how the children are doing are put on a back-burner during the period of marital therapy. Sometimes I think that it is very easy to collude with the parents and forget about the children. Sometimes it takes a little bit of assertiveness or perseverance on the part of the therapist to be fairly incisive and inquire specifically about the children during this period of marital distress. These are situations where the parents are not defining the children as having any symptoms. The second response to your question is, I always ask couples, not always in the first visit but perhaps in the second or third visit, what have they told their children about coming to see me and, as you know, many couples have not told their children anything.

I have also been struck by the fact that many couples want some sort of guidance from the therapist on this issue. They may not ask directly about it but I do respond to it directly. My general feeling is that I like parents to inform their children, so that they know mom and dad are going off to see Dr. X, whom the children have not met at this time, once a week for a period of time. I've learned that one the hard way by my experience with one of my former patients who was divorced. About three years after the divorce, she told me that her daughter asked her one day, "Why didn't you and daddy go for marital help when you were having so many problems?" Her mother said, "Well, we did, we saw Dr. X." Her daughter burst into tears at that point and looked her in the eye and said, "If you would only have told me, I would have felt that you were trying to do something about it." I guess the message is that the daughter had no thought that the parents were actually trying to do something about their marital distress. My third response to the question is that if I'm ever sufficiently concerned or if I'm told that the parents are ignoring the children, then I do request at least one family visit. When a decision to separate has been made and the family is in the process of doing so physically, I almost always see the entire family so that I can talk with the kids about some of the normal strains and stresses associated with separation.

Comment: I'm glad to hear that. I think we tend to think that here is the parents' marriage at a low point when they have children and here the children are being exposed to the parents at the low point in their marriage—it is a two-way street. I can remember seeing a bumper sticker once when I was in court or someplace that said that mental illness was hereditary, you get it from your children. I think we really have to keep in mind—looking through the telescope from the other end.

Question: I found your talk very interesting, but it seemed to me that you have raised a couple of points that need clarification. The assessment procedures and ways of dealing with motivation of marital couples in crisis seemed to me slightly different than when one is embarking on longer-term therapies. In fact, maybe a lot more than slightly. I think it would make it very difficult to have a set pattern of intervention when different situations call for different modes of involvement of the therapist. I wondered if there was a possibility that you could expand on that.

Answer: This is a good point. I agree completely with you, in a crisis situation I am more often taking my cues from the individuals rather than from the couple itself as to where to go next and sort of getting a reading on them each week. If, for instance, there is extreme distress, and provided there is no violence or threat of violence and one partner is feeling pretty hopeless about the relationship and wants to separate, I try and get them to stall on that if possible and to give me an opportunity to have four conjoint visits with them. After these visits, I hope they will be better able to make the decision whether separation is indeed the correct choice. Most times people are able to come to that kind of agreement.

Comment: To follow that up, it seems to me that in this sort of situation one might legitimately borrow from crisis intervention techniques in terms of when one gets involved with individuals. As we go beyond these techniques, it seems to me that we get into the challenge of trying to understand the dynamics of relationships that affect communication and intimacy, power sharing, and so forth.

Question: There seems to be a gap between what we as therapists do, which is to use multiple models and multiple techniques in the service of flexibility. Almost everybody who has spoken this morning has indicated that they favor flexibility and using a number of different models. Dr. Waring suggested that the model to help us understand married couples cannot be so reductionistic as to be something that was used to explain the behavior of rats. Dr. Martin said earlier today that he thinks most people who are experienced therapists are quite eclectic, even more so than they admit. On the other hand, we have heard everybody saying that there is a need for more research and if you look at the research, there is a lot of specificity. Techniques have to have specificity to meet the criteria for research. How do we deal with this? I wonder if you have a sense of this problem. You were talking in a language that would indicate to me that you are a very flexible therapist. You not only use multiple techniques, but you have a definite notion that marital therapy is something that may be considered part of an overall therapeutic approach. You also have respect for the marital life cycle, so please tell us how can we learn more in terms of specific research if we are also using such flexible and multiple techniques.

Answer: I have a lot of difficulty even with questionnaires, although I do use them for certain couples. These are questionnaires that I use to obtain data on unmet needs in each partner. For some couples they are very helpful. Also, it is sometimes very useful for each of the spouses to share that information. To reply to your question, I really don't know. Recently I sat in on a presentation given by a behaviorist who was well known in marital therapy, and where all of the behavioral expectations were very neatly drawn up. I had a lot of trouble even listening to that paper. I found myself getting a knot in my stomach. I asked a question and it came out so hostile that I even surprised myself. The question had something to do with, "Does anybody listen to the patient?"

Comment: I just wanted to respond a little bit to that comment. I think this is an interesting issue for the field of marital therapy. While it is good to try to clarify our concepts and operationalize them and try to research them as much as possible, I think we have to accept the nature of the beast: marital distress is not something that lends itself to research as easily as other fields of endeavor. Something that I think is rampant in psychiatry in general, and also in marital therapy, is a certain kind of physics envy. We want to be able to measure and quantify, and be able to do things that may be unrealistic. The time is ripe now because of the more humanistic approach that Dr. Waring was referring to earlier. Research is another issue; it is good, indeed it can't be bad, but it is so difficult. I think that is why when you look at anything that has been researched you find so many different answers.

Question: I wanted to respond to a few things you said. Each one of those three models is appropriate and is true and valid. There are also neurotics in London! Part of us has been evolutionarily related to rats! I think that what makes marriages different or what makes an enduring heterosexual relationship different is an important question. I think there are a lot of assumptions underlying your ideas of marriage that I can dispute because I don't think that intimacy is necessarily a marital goal in most of the world. I know that when I teach people about marriage in a city as heterogeneous as Montreal, how am I going to start expecting marital intimacy from an Italian or Greek couple, when the whole question of what is important or what the malignant forces are that you describe, Dr. Rosenbluth, is so different. One of the things that wasn't mentioned as "a malignant force" in marriages is the extended family and their expectations and pressures and the loyalty problems involved. I think that one of our problems is that even if we want to look at marriage as an enduring heterosexual relationship, we have to look at it within the context of the tremendous number of cultural values and expectations and ideas, even about heterosexuality and what that means. I would like to ask Dr. Myers a question. You talked about switching modalities and I wonder how you do that so readily? What are some of the indications that you would have in a crisis situation for switching between the modalities of marital therapy—that is certainly something that I have a lot of difficulty understanding.

Answer: I was thinking more that I switch from a conjoint format to an individual concurrent model. I find that if after two or three conjoint visits that it is not working then there may be some block. Then I will shift focus and explain to the spouses why I would continue with them each individually again.

Question: You've never had situations where you feel that your type of therapy is not the appropriate type for that particular couple.

Answer: Oh, sure.

Question: What do you do then?

Answer: You mean if I feel that the type of therapy just isn't working for the couple?

Question: No, I don't know how to do behavioral marriage

therapy. I really don't know how to do it. I might think it was appropriate, but I don't know how to do it.

Answer: Okay, I wasn't talking about behavioral marriage therapy in a very sophisticated way. I'm talking about things like encouraging the spouses to go out one night in the next week together outside of the home so that they can have a 2-hour conversation about this particular visit. If they come back the following week without having done that then we can talk about it so I get a sense of their behavioral resistance. If it has to do with one person trying to change an item of behavior, then I would try to have the other partner work on changing an item of behavior simultaneously.

Question: I have seen people from all sorts of ethnic and cultural backgrounds, and it is interesting that I have not yet seen a Chinese couple, despite the large Chinese population. I don't know why but I would be interested to know. I think the similarities and the differences in marriage are very similar, irrespective of the couple's cultural background. Often cultural background is brought in, in a sense, to explain away the spouses' aberrant behavior but this is really a screen and is quite easily dealt with. I think the basic issue is the partners' capacity for intimacy. I wouldn't agree that intimacy is not an issue in other cultures. I think that is a kind of Western myth.

Dr. Waring: I would address this issue in a different way. I think there is a difference between studying the interpersonal psychological variables of intimacy in any two-person relationship and claiming, which we don't, that people consciously marry in order to develop intimacy. Nobody does that! At least, very few people do that. The fact that we go out to the general population and find that 15 percent of the population has optimal intimacy, as we operationally define it, doesn't mean that that is a cherished value for those people and is why they got married in the first place. They didn't get married for those reasons at all. The same observation applies to people who have a very low level of intimacy. In other cultures and in our culture, couples stay in their relationships because the motives for the relationship are totally different from the psychological and interpersonal motives. They are staying together for socioeconomic reasons, or for other kinds of reasons.

Question: You see, I would fundamentally disagree with you. I think that in any culture there are different dimensions of intimacy and individuals seek them via relationships with different people. The first statement you made was that the most important relationship is the husband–wife relationship.

Dr. Waring: No, what I said is that's what we found in these optimally intimate couples that we studied here in London. Exactly right, that is what *they* say. That is not true across the board and most of those relationships are only functional.

Question: I think as therapists we have to guard against these kinds of preconceptions in order to be effective.

Dr. Waring: Michael is saying that the treatment isn't designed for people who say they are there in order to have Bill not go out and play baseball with the boys on Friday nights. This couple's treatment would not necessarily be designed to facilitate their intimacy, it would be designed to keep Bill from playing baseball on Friday night!

Answer: I just want to add a different dimension to the intimacy argument. I think that when we are talking about intimacy and also research on intimacy over the past decade, we think of the couples we have seen in our own practices. I wonder how many of us sitting here have come from homes where their parents went for marital therapy or even considered it. I wonder whether it was even available because the type of marriage is changing. When you look at the demography of marriages it is quite fascinating how some years ago (I wouldn't know exactly how many) in some of the Quebec research it was more common that one spouse would die before the last child had left home. Well, nowadays the figures show that the couple are going to be living together 20 years after that last child leaves. In the older model the spouses died off before they really had to come to grips with each other, and in Western culture marriages are supposed to be for companionship or love, whereas in other cultures they are more for economic reasons, and so on.

Question: I think there is some cultural component. I come from a background where my father never so much as spoke to my mother until they were married and they never held hands until the marriage, yet it was a total commitment. Love and sexuality grow out of mutual commitment on the part of the husband and wife, whereas in occidental cultures many people marry for better or worse, but not for good!

Chapter 6

MARITAL THERAPY:
Outcome Research—Multiple Pathways to Progress

Paul M. Cameron

Holt[1] has stated: "One of the first and most fundamental problems of experimental research in clinical psychology is how to discipline observations so that questions can be answered with some degree of confidence without abandoning commitment to answer humanly important questions."

The study of therapeutic intervention and outcome with respect to marital and sexual life is a vital and humanly important question. Marital satisfaction is crucial to the quality of life, to the prevention of mental stress and disorder, and to shaping the psychological and social development of children.

Prevention strategies demand more of our attention and

Many thanks to Ms. Joan Kemp for her valuable assistance in preparing this chapter.

more research funding in present-day psychiatry. Philips[2] summarizes opportunities for us to develop prevention strategies: reducing marital distress, facilitating separation and divorce, and recognizing high-risk children among the offspring of parents with major psychiatric diseases such as affective disorder.

According to Sager demand for marital therapy is increasing,[3] yet few training programs in psychiatry offer adequate training in marital therapy.[4]

This chapter will focus on three broad themes in the marital therapy outcome literature:

1. Evidence concerning effectiveness of marital therapy.
2. The crucial problems in methodology and in the conceptualization of research directed at the outcome of marital therapy, along with some current strategies to solve these problems.
3. Different pathways that may lead to further progress in our understanding of marital therapy process and outcome.

The central thesis of this chapter is that pursuing multiple pathways directed at answering specific questions will yield varied information that will improve the impact of our interventions and will help us design relevant new hypotheses for future research.

EFFECTIVENESS

Gurman and Kniskern[5] report the following global improvement rates in their review of two hundred studies of marital and family therapy:

Nonbehavioral marital therapy   61 percent improved
Behavioral marital therapy   64 percent improved

Masters and Johnson,[6] Kaplan,[7] and Gurman and Kniskern[5] put the following rates of improvement for common sexual dysfunctions. These are:

Primary orgasmic dysfunction	90 percent improved
Secondary orgasmic dysfunction	50 percent improved
Premature ejaculation	90 percent improved
Primary erectile failure	50 percent improved
Secondary erectile failure	70 percent improved

These rates of improvement seem quite high. Why is there such controversy in the field? Any comment on psychotherapy research needs to address the basic challenge of Eysenck[8,9] and Rachman[10] who claim that psychotherapy techniques that are nonbehavioral have not been proven to be more effective than spontaneous remission rates in untreated neurotic patients. Bergin and Lambert[11] have reviewed these claims and have demonstrated them to be false based on the following findings. Eysenck and Rachman have considered only part of the available data that support their claims in favor of behavioral techniques. Eysenck made errors in calculation and recording of data in that he demanded more rigorous criteria for improvement in psychotherapy than he used for his claims of spontaneous recovery in 66 percent of untreated patients. To substantiate his claim of a high rate of spontaneous recovery in patients who had not had psychotherapy, he relied on disability insurance studies. The population of patients treated and those apparently recovered without treatment were not shown to be similar.

However, this polarized debate continues and contaminates much of the marital therapy research literature as well as the literature on individual psychotherapy. Gurman and Kniskern[5] point out that spontaneous improvement in marital disorder has not been demonstrated to be as high as 66 percent. Bergin and Lambert[11] suggest that spontaneous recovery in untreated individuals may in fact be as low as 30 percent. Malan, Bacal, et al.[12] have shown that some patients thought to be spontaneously recovering have sought other therapeutic encounters while on psychotherapy waiting lists, and that some patients receive benefit from extremely brief assessment interviews.

My own training and orientation should be stated explicitly in order to allow readers to examine both my clinical experience and my theoretical bias. I have received 2 years of training in marital and family therapy, 2 years of training in behavioral therapy and psychotherapy research, and 4 years of training in psychoanalysis. For 18 years I have employed all three modes of psychotherapy, singly and in combination, attempting to tailor the treatment techniques to my formulation of the patient's or couple's clinical situation.[13, 14]

My theoretical perspective is that *some patients require multiple techniques*[15] to achieve maximum relief of symptoms and to develop their full capacity to enjoy the maximum quality of life. This is true for attainment of full marital, sexual, and occupational satisfaction.

There are other patients or couples, however, who may achieve *entirely adequate improvement with only one technique*. It is also likely that there is more than one pathway to produce improvement in some patients. They can be treated with either behavioral or dynamic or cognitive therapy. Our knowledge base needs to improve so that we can identify which patients require which interventions and in what sequence.

One more general psychotherapy study may help us to appreciate much of the highly polarized debate in the literature. A recent study by Smith, Glass, and Miller[16] examined 475 control studies of many forms of psychotherapy including marital therapy. The conclusion these authors reached is that psychotherapy produces an overall improvement rate greater than most interventions that have been described in the social sciences. The conclusions are based on a technique described as *meta-analysis*, which is a statistical analysis of the outcome data that examines the effect of change or improvement in the treatment group compared to control groups or comparison groups.

The patient who is in the 50th percentile at baseline will at the end of psychotherapy be better off than 80 percent of those who need therapy but remain untreated. These authors conclude that behavioral techniques produce more improvement than nonbehavioral or dynamic therapies. Such a conclusion is made by many groups in the field although there are contradictory opinions such as those of Gurman and Kniskern[5] who suggested that the different rates of improvement, particularly in marital therapy, are small and subject to interpretation. Opinions differ markedly with respect to the significance of change reported to result from many different techniques. This chapter will often refer to this tension between the advocates of behavioral and nonbehavioral therapy, but I hope to demonstrate that both approaches have value. The question to be asked, is, "For what patients and in what sequences can these approaches be combined or used separately? When is one technique both necessary and sufficient?"

EFFECTIVENESS OF DIFFERENT TECHNIQUES

Gurman and Kniskern[5] suggest the following overall improvement rates for different techniques:

Conjoint marital therapy	65 percent improvement
Individual psychotherapy for marital disorder	48 percent improvement

Combing conjoint therapy with individual sessions may often be useful for certain patients. Studies comparing conjoint therapy to conjoint group therapy produce no difference in improvement rates. Conjoint therapy is superior to no treatment or control groups in 10 of 15 studies.

Behavioral marital therapy techniques are very popular and, as in individual psychotherapy, they are very effective if the correct technique is selected for a suitable patient. The goals of behavioral marital therapy are to increase the rate of pleasing and rewarding interaction and decrease the rate of aversive or displeasing interaction. The teaching of concrete conflict resolution techniques and problem-solving skills, as well as improving communication skills, are common features. Certain observable behaviors are rated on a self-report checklist and identified as either pleasing or displeasing. This allows the development of a contingency schedule where both members of the couple agree on which behaviors are to be increased and which behaviors are to be decreased. Various instruments or checklists are available to record data in various categories.

Some of these measurement instruments include the Locke-Wallace Marital Adjustment Scale,[17] the Spouse Observation Check List (SOC),[18] and the Marital Interaction Coding System.[19]

- In 7 of 11 studies behavioral marital therapy produce more improvement than no treatment.
- In 8 of 16 studies behavioral marital therapy produced more improvement than comparison treatments.

There is overwhelming evidence that behavioral marital therapy techniques are effective in changing certain observable behaviors, and in particular there is much agreement that some of the communication skills packages available are very useful.[20, 21]

Difficulties in interpreting the meaningfulness and the specific indications for behavioral therapy techniques constitute critical problems with this type of therapy. Crowe[22] has indicated that behavioral techniques are often resisted by couples who have a high level of education and are from the upper and upper-middle social classes. This has been confirmed by my own clinical experience.

A more technical problem is that the search for measures that demonstrate improvement due to change in behavioral therapy techniques raises important questions. It is possible to question whether couples are reporting the most significant type of change and improvement for them in terms of preserving the overall quality of their marital bond, or whether they are merely reporting that they have changed behaviors that they have been trained to change. Often the evaluation of improvement focuses more on the latter than on other less behavioral measures. This matter will be discussed in more detail under Methodological Problems and Conceptual Issues (p. 114), where I will focus on how to determine whether a couple has improved. A final reservation about the enthusiasm with which behavioral marital therapy techniques are being advocated as being superior to other techniques is that there is no adequate evidence, according to Jacobson and Martin[23] regarding the relative importance of each component of these techniques. However, further progress is very likely possible as a result of marital therapy techniques because they are in fact observable, teachable, replicable, measurable, and specific.

DETERIORATION RATES

Patients deteriorate in marital therapy, that is, they may report more distress, develop new problems, and feel that the overall quality of their relationship is worse at the end of treatment than it was before treatment. Separation and divorce occur but cannot always be seen as merely a negative effect, since this may be a desirable outcome. Between 5 and 10 percent of couples in marital therapy will have a negative outcome. With regard to people in individual therapy for marital problems, negative outcome is reflected in an even higher 11.6 percent deterioration rate. However, this may be due to the selection of couples placed in that treatment modality; these spouses may demonstrate either ambivalence with regard to the fate of the relationship or significant character pathology that may be more likely to lead to separation and divorce. Couples who are offered individual treatment for marital problems often do not demonstrate *momentum* as described by Rosenbluth and Cameron.[24] It is not clear yet whether lack of willingness and ability to move forward to work on problems is always a powerful obstacle to conjoint therapy. However, Kaplan in her book on sexual therapy[7] suggests that many characteristics similar to the concept of momentum are necessary for sexual therapy to demonstrate positive results, and Kaplan indicates that often the presence of lack of momentum in its various forms is an indication for marital therapy in addition to sex therapy.

OTHER FACTORS INFLUENCING OUTCOME

These are variables located in the patients, the process of treatment, and the therapist.

Patient Variables

Severity of disorder or chronicity of distress correlates negatively with outcome[25] although there are contradictory studies to this trend.

Husbands have a key role to play in the outcome of therapy. First, they are expected by their wives not to be willing to attend—an expectation that often proves to be false. When they do attend, if they are the identified patient, the outcome is more positive.[26] Men respond differently to marital therapy when combined with sex therapy as shown by Hartmann[26] and report improvement in sexual enjoyment more in response to marital therapy than sex therapy. Self acceptance of sexual enjoyment is more effectively accomplished by marital therapy. However, sexual therapy helped males understand their mates better. These observations raised the complicated question of whether marital and sexual therapy need to be combined, and, if so, in what sequence or for which couples. A detailed discussion of this issue is found in Kaplan.[7]

Mendonca, Lumley, and Hunt[27] show that only the husband's traits correlated significantly with improvement in their study, particularly with respect to improvement in affective communication. Important traits were the husband's cognitive skill, reflection and judgment, submissiveness, and sensitivity to social approval of his behavior.

Educational differences affect outcome. If the husband has more education than his wife, this difference favorably effects the outcome according to Freeman and coauthors[28] and Wattie.[29] Crowe[22] also found that higher educated couples do better with interpretive psychotherapy than with direct behavioral measures.

Beck and Jones[25] found that male therapists were more often able to keep the husband in treatment; however, female patients terminated earlier with male therapists compared to female patients who had female therapists.

Wives improve more in marital therapy if they receive individual sessions according to Mendonca and coauthors.[27] Hartmann[26] found that sex therapy produced greater improvement in sexual enjoyment when used in conjunction with marital therapy for females. Mothers who are good decision makers have more favorable outcomes according to Bowen.[30]

Family interaction studies are very common and seem to yield some useful prediction information, which is sadly needed in this field. Couples stay in treatment if they are low on authoritarianism,[31] open to disagreement, and are less coercive and competitive.[32]

Spouse-spouse attitude convergence is a more important predictor of outcome than spouse-therapist attitude convergence according to Gurman.[5] Couples of low socioeconomic status usually require different techniques, with emphasis on direct advice.

Therapist Variables

Experienced therapists effect more positive outcomes;[28,35] however, other studies report no difference.[36] Cotherapy may be a more enjoyable and effective process but there is no evidence of its superiority in outcome. In fact, a negative correlation might occur if the experience difference level of the cotherapists is high.[34] The gender of the therapist is not clearly related to outcome although the McMaster Group suggested that the male therapist has a better outcome.[36] The authors claim this finding held for patient ratings but did not remain constant for objective measures of outcome.

An important therapist variable is relationship skill or the capacity to develop a therapeutic alliance. We know that such a capacity is important in all forms of psychotherapy. Hollis[39] claimed that therapist involvement as measured by activity, empathy, and catharsis, rather than quiet reflectiveness, is positively correlated with outcome. Guttman, Sigal, Epstein, and Postner[40] rated the quality of therapist interventions and showed that therapists' direct statements, as compared with therapists' interpretive statements, are those that simulate interaction, give support, or collect information, whereas therapists' interpretive statements have to do with clarifying motivation or labeling unconscious motivation. Therapists' interpretive statements are viewed as primarily onus-putting and anxiety-provoking. Three-quarters of the families studied dropped out early and prematurely if there was a low D/I ratio, meaning that there was more interpretive (I) than direct (D) forms of intervention. The conclusion these authors reached was that a high interpretive rate of interventions is too confronting or onus-putting for some families. In 1976, Alexander and coworkers[41] showed that relationship skill, which he described as expression of warmth, affective behavior, interpretation, and humor accounted for 45 percent of the variability regarding the success of therapy outcome, whereas technical skills only accounted for 15 percent. Presumably, client and process variables were responsible for the remaining 40 percent of success variability.

The length of treatment is an important issue in this field. Time-limited treatment does not appear to be inferior to open-ended or longer-term treatment. This is a common statement that applies to all forms of psychotherapy. I believe it is too simplistic. Reid and Shyne[42] showed that couples with 8 sessions of marital therapy had better outcomes than with 26, and that husbands do better with fewer sessions. It is likely true that the marriages of many couples can be improved significantly with 10 to 20 sessions of marital therapy; however, it is also likely true that there are a number of couples who require more treatment than this and that they should not be deprived of the treatment. It is necessary to carefully study the residual effects at the end of treatment and try to define a subpopulation that requires more assistance. In Crowe's[22] careful outcome study, it was found that 15 of his 42 couples requested further treatment, more than the 5 to 10 sessions offered. He also found that a number of these patients had a higher level of education and were seeking an interpretive type of treatment rather than a behavioral one.

METHODOLOGICAL PROBLEMS AND CONCEPTUAL ISSUES

Nosology, Diagnosis, and Classification in Marital Dysfunction

Berman and Lief[43] pointed out in their creative paper, "Marital Therapy from a Psychiatric Perspective: An Overview," that there is no comprehensive or consensual classifications system or typology of marital disorder. Martin[4] and others have suggested some classifications focusing on qualities of the object relationship or on certain characterologic features, and the interaction between these two aspects. However, there is no agreed convention whereby one may accept any system that accurately and reliably describes homogeneous populations. Therefore, diagnostic research criteria facilitating comparison of studies do not exist.

Subclassifications

Medical illness. Some early signs of a solution are appearing. Specific populations are being described and specific marital therapy techniques are being suggested. For instance, couples with medical illness require specific approaches[44] and specific syndromes are being studied such as conjoint therapy involving myocardial infarction patients,[45] and postmastectomy groups with spouses.[47]

Major psychiatric illness. Couples in which one member is suffering from a major psychiatric disorder such as alcoholism and major affective disorders are also described separately because they require specific techniques when the affected spouse is also involved in treatment.

Most couples presenting to therapists demonstrate marital conflicts, sexual problems, and some difficulty to do wih character structure that prevents or interferes with intimacy and other aspects of a satisfying mutual relationship. These dysfunctions are difficult to subclassify. The DSM-III has attempted to classify some forms of character disorder although there is not widespread agreement that the methods used are the best possible ones according to Robert Michels[48] and Livesely, who are also studying the validity of this system.[49]

I suggest that we need to attempt to describe different subpopulations of this group by first excluding other groups mentioned above, such as those individuals with serious medical illnesses, or serious psychiatric disorders. Then, carefully using and critically evaluating the DSM-III classification and other diagnostic systems, we need to build an experience of treating this population while attempting to describe subgroups within it. There are various instruments to help us measure qualities of the marital relationship such as Olson's Pair Inventory[50] or Warings Intimacy Questionnaire.[51] Both these instruments have been validated on clinical and nonclinical populations.

Excessive Adherence to Particular School of Therapy or Psychopathology

Gurman and Kniskern[5] and many others lament this problem that confounds the literature. The GAP Report on family conflict in 1975[52] suggested that despite doctrinaire differences, some concensus could be developed enabling a core battery of instruments for measuring change to be put together. This promise has not been fulfilled yet. In Canada we may be well situated to achieve this because we tend not to attach ourselves to charismatic leaders and doctrinaire schools of thought as much as some other parts of the psychiatric community. In other areas of psychiatry, such as development of learning objectives in psychiatric residency education, we have benefited by less polarization and emphasis on genuine eclecticism on the part of rival schools within our academic departments of psychiatry.

Research Design

Many issues have prevented us from making progress on what seems to be a manageable problem. After all, why, in the face of significant effectiveness in global ratings, can we not dissect the techniques and patient-therapist process variables that either maximize or minimize improvement? Here are some of the obstacles:

Selection of criteria to measure change (either improvement or deterioration). This is a crucial problem in all psychotherapy research. Parloff[53] in a National Institute of Mental Health (NIMH) report, suggested a core battery of tests may be possible for individual psychotherapy research. Changes must be assessed at multiple levels including both external and internal changes. There is some agreement on the different levels that need to be tested, although the vast number of instruments for testing require some decisions to be made about which instruments may be most useful. However, the levels for testing are:

1. Self-concept, examining self-esteem, autonomy.
2. Perception of the relationship using intimacy questionnaires or marital satisfaction questionnaires.
3. A symptom checklist, such as the General Health Questionnaire (GHQ).
4. Specific dynamic target symptoms.
5. Behavioral measures, either reported or observed in sessions or in simulated situations.
6. Social, occupational, and leisure relationship inventory as developed by Gurland.[54]
7. Family issues regarding parenting and family interaction systems.

Most of these levels are used by Crowe[22] in one of the more carefully controlled studies in the field. Of course this study is not without weaknesses and can be criticized, but it has addressed this issue relatively well.

Agreement on how to measure these levels of function and with what instruments, and to offer further follow-

up to certain selective cases. Gurman and Kniskern[5] point out that there are well over one hundred instruments and often the instruments used are related to the theoretical orientation of the researchers. It seems that the only way of dealing with this is to use at least some instruments that include the two major orientations—the behavioral and psychodynamic schools.

Change is multidimensional. Gurman and Kniskern[5] suggests that divergent processes occur in therapeutic change and divergent methods of criterion measurement must therefore be used to capture these changes. We also have a problem interpreting improvement and change if there is a difference on some measures. How do we know what is important enough improvement for the couple? Can we rely on their self-reports alone? Woodward and Santa-Barbara[38] would suggest that this is not wise since they point out that there is much divergence in the manner couples, treated in their center, rate their satisfaction with treatment.

Individually tailored criteria of change. Specific goals need to be individualized. This is a widely accepted orientation in psychotherapy research. Malan[55] in 1976 developed specific dynamic hypotheses that can be rated with interrater reliability. These hypotheses will not only tailor the outcome of the individual patient, but will anticipate their level of coping in future situations. Battle, Imber, and Frank[56] developed a target complaint scale in 1966, and a goal attainment scale was developed by Kiresuk and Shurman[57] in 1968. All are useful approaches to this problem.

Multiple rating perspectives. Most studies reported in Gurman and Kniskern's review up to 1978[5] used only global ratings and were heavily weighted to rely exclusively on clients' reports. Clearly this is inadequate although it may have some value in a naturalistic study for the purpose of clinical audit of one's own practice. However, to advance the field one needs to have client and therapist-blind independent raters and, if possible, information from significant others. Crowe[22] has managed to do this in his study.

What is enough improvement? If different measures show different rates of change and if different raters have disagreement in the amount of change they note, how do we decide what weight to give the many aspects of the multidimensional improvement or changed profile? Woodward and coauthors[38] reported that consumer satisfaction is not correlated with improvement in a family therapy service in a large McMaster clinic* treating 270 families. In her study in 1978, 45 percent of families were dissatisfied with the comprehensive inadequacy of the service, 68 percent said that they were generally satisfied with the experience, and 79 percent were feeling better about most of their original problems. One may bypass these concerns of the validity of self-reports by setting up objective measures. However, the question could be asked whether the presence of significant improvement in objective measures can be a meaningful finding when the couple states that they are dissatisfied. This is a complex problem and I don't have an immediate solution, but more dialogue should be encouraged to examine what truly heavily weighted outcome measures seem to exist across many studies. Surely one must listen to the patient's self-reports but we need to put in their hands the most effective instruments to communicate their self-evaluation.

Control Groups. Few studies have dealt with the no-

---

* The McMaster University Clinic in Hamilton, Ontario uses a McMaster model of family therapy developed by N. B. Epstein and researched by C. Woodward and coworkers. It is also researched now at Brown University by Epstein and Bishop.

treatment control group well. The study of Candy, Marks, Malan et al.[58] has dealt with some of the severe ethical, referral, and design problems when long-term psychotherapy studies require a no-treatment control group. I was associated with this study for 2 years and agreed with the conclusion that to study long-term psychotherapy in an ideal fashion is not feasible. This does not mean that long-term psychotherapy, individual or marital, is not indicated as the treatment of choice for some couples, but it helps to explain the trend toward the briefer research studies.

One way of maintaining perspective in this matter would be to honestly face this question: If oneself or one's close relative or child was in marital distress, would you send that person to five to 10 sessions of a prepackaged behavioral treatment alone without considering other aspects of their distress? Ironically, most people in the mental health field do not seek such treatment for themselves on this basis, yet they may participate in studies with a reductionistic approach because such studies are possible to design and execute.

Dimascio and Klerman in 1977 developed the treatment on demand of control groups in psychotherapy research (personal communication). This mode of treatment makes it possible to solve some of the problems, especially with briefer therapeutic strategies.

What are all the necessary features of an adequate outcome study in terms of research design? As we would expect, there is controversy here. In 1979 Gale[59] suggested that there were no adequate studies in the literature. Gurman and Kniskern[5] disagree and rate approximately 60 studies of marital therapy, over half of which they evaluate as good or very good. They suggest 14 criteria for an excellent study based on outcome. These criteria are:

1. Controlled assignment to treatment conditions.

2. Pre- and post-study measurement of change.
3. No contamination of major independent variables including therapist experience level and relevant therapeutic competence.
4. Appropriate statistical analysis.
5. Follow-up in excess of 3 months.
6. Treatments equally valued.
7. Treatment carried out as described or expected and evidence to support this.
8. Multiple change indices.
9. Multiple vantage points to assess outcome.
10. Outcome not limited to change in the identified patient.
11. Data on other concurrent treatments.
12. Equal treatment length to compare the studies.
13. Outcome assessment measures for positive and negative change.
14. A therapist-investigator nonequivalence (investigator should not be a therapist).

Gurman and Kniskern rated studies on these 14 criteria in a manner described in their paper and concluded that there was a significant number of good and worthwhile studies with conclusions with which I agree. Frude,[60] however, argues that we must consider the real-world clinical situation when we design studies. He favored Lask's[61] more simple demands of an acceptable study.

1. The independent variable should be a clear definition of a treatment used, which should consist predominantly of conjoint interviews.
2. Families should be randomly assigned to experimental and control groups.
3. The two groups should be matched in all important variables.
4. There must be a clear definition of all outcome measures used.

5. The follow-up period should be adequate.

Frude's[60] practical notions about the viewpoint of the clinician advance the possibility that there may be a useful dialogue between clinicians and researchers. He points out that purists such as Gale[59] insist on such complexity of design that studies they design may be nonfeasible. Many different forms of research design will offer different types of information but it is foolish to discard any of the proven types of research. We can learn from naturalistic studies describing our own practices as we may participate in such studies without having to change our current techniques or reduce them. We can learn from experimental or analog designs that look at certain aspects of family interaction using decision-making tasks. Obviously, we certainly can learn from control or comparative studies and we can learn from multidimensional and multicenter studies as well. Lastly, we can learn from negative reports. Even experienced clinicians such as Rakoff, Sigal, and Epstein[62] reporting their negative results with regard to their ability to predict outcome, lead us to useful hypotheses and cause us to consider soberly some of our own assumptions. Interestingly, in this study patients often rated their outcome as being more successful than did their therapists.

In 1978, Marks[63] suggested that no research effort can answer all or most questions with one grand multifactoral study. It is more feasible to consider designing a program of smaller studies that deals with a specific set of research questions. Marks also suggested that a good lesson for a research student to learn is that each experimental design can answer only a very few questions. The selection of any particular research design precludes answering many other questions.

MULTIPLE PATHWAYS TO MORE EFFECTIVE INTERVENTIONS

We have observed that there is considerable evidence that psychotherapy for marital disorder is globally effective in 67 percent of couples but that 5 to 12 percent of couples may deteriorate. Up to 20 percent of couples may drop out of therapy. This figure can be higher with some of the behavioral techniques. Individual psychotherapy for marital problems is said to have a lower success rate of 48 percent. However, this may include couples for whom individual therapy is the most appropriate treatment because they are headed inevitably toward separation and divorce. A means of assessing momentum as a way of selecting a treatment modality would be useful.[24]

There are multiple pathways by which we can learn new information that will provide us with heuristic hypotheses. The evidence favors using studies designed specifically to answer certain questions, using a specific population, in line with the comments of Marks[63] and Frude[60] who believe each type of research strategy has information to offer. A particular type of study should not be criticized from a destructive point of view simply because it does not emphasize a certain investigator's bias. For example, one may easily view Crowe's[22] 1978 study as a careful and interesting attempt, one of the first studies to assign 42 couples randomly to a behavioral technique, an interpretive technique, and a minimum-contact support technique. It is easy to praise the number of measures of outcome, the number of vantage points, and the cautiousness of the conclusions.

A more critical review would highlight the many limitations of Crowe's study:

- Fifteen of the 42 couples wished further treatment. What does this imply about the design of the study?
- The interpretive therapy did *not* employ transference, unconscious motivation, or any linkages with parents or the nuclear family. Crowe states that expressed enthusiasm is only an integral part of direct behavioral treatment, *not* of the interpretive treatment. He uses this position as evidence that if recordings monitored his treatments and found that

he was enthusiastic for behavioral treatment, this would prove that he was doing good behavioral therapy and that his interpretive technique was different and more relevant to interpretive techniques in general. Many would question whether purposely restraining enthusiasm would be a valid form of using interpretive techniques.

It could also be argued that combining interpretive techniques with behavioral techniques would have resulted in a more useful comparison group since this is likely to be a much more common approach to marital therapy.

In conclusion let me make the following points:

1. We advocate that different investigations can yield specific contributions that are quite different. Authors who are attempting to integrate the evidence that is accumulating with regard to marital therapy outcome and those who are designing new studies must be able to accept that there are currently *multiple pathways* for the effective treatment of couples.

2. Research strategies, too, can be viewed as multiple pathways to adding certain specific types of information to the total information pool.

3. Our training programs need to produce flexible professional therapists who can utilize more than one technique and who are aware of the developing body of information that points to specific populations and recommends specific techniques.

4. Based on the available evidence it appears that there are a number of couples who require *multiple therapeutic modalities* to fully treat their range of symptoms. Kaplan,[7] Gurman,[5] and Hartmann[26] provide us with evidence for this hypothesis.

5. It is also likely that there are many subpopulations

of couples who can be treated equally as well using different techniques. This would confirm much of the psychotherapy research literature.

6. Finally, there are likely certain subpopulations of couples who *need* a *particular technique* and may not receive such treatment if the clinician involved is not able to make the proper formulation and select from the full range of techniques available. Genuine eclecticism and collaboration will advance this complex field more than doctrinaire and reductionistic polarization. Continuing dialogue between investigators and therapists using different techniques, singly and in combination, will enrich the appreciation of all therapists with regard to the options available for their patients.

REFERENCES

1. Holt, R. (1965). Experimental methods in clinical psychology. In B. Wolman (Ed.), *Handbook of clinical psychology* (p. 44). New York: McGraw-Hill.
2. Philips, I. (1983). Opportunities for prevention in the practice of psychiatry. *American Journal of Psychiatry, 140*(4):389–396.
3. Sager, C. (1976). *Marriage contracts and couple therapy.* New York: Brunner/Mazel.
4. Martin, P. (1976). *A marital therapy manual.* New York: Brunner/Mazel.
5. Gurman, A., & Kniskern, D. (1978). Research on marital and family therapy. In H. Bergin & S. Garfield (Eds.), *Handbook of psychotherapy and behavior change* (2nd ed.) New York: John Wiley & Sons.
6. Master, W., & Johnson, V. (1970). *Human sexual inadequacy.* Boston: Little, Brown.
7. Kaplan, H. S. (1974). *The new sex therapy.* New York: Brunner/Mazel.
8. Eysenck, H. J. (1952). The effects of psychotherapy: An evaluation. *Journal of Consulting Psychology, 16,* 319–324.
9. Eysenck, H. J. (1966). *The effects of psychotherapy.* New York: International Science Press.
10. Rachman, S. (1971). *The effects of psychotherapy.* Oxford: Pergamon Press.

11. Bergin, A. E., & Lambert, M. (1978). The evaluation of therapeutic outcomes. In H. Bergin & S. Garfield (Eds.), *Handbook of psychotherapy and behavior change* (2nd ed.). New York: John Wiley & Sons.
12. Malan, D., Bacal, H., et al. (1975). Psychodynamic changes in unrelated subjects. *Archives of General Psychiatry, 32,* 110–126.
13. Cameron, P. M., Kline, S. A., et al. (1978). A method of reporting formulation. *Canadian Psychiatric Association Journal, 23,* 43–50.
14. Kline, S. A., & Cameron, P. M. (1978). Formulation. *Canadian Psychiatric Association Journal, 23,* 39–43.
15. Cameron, P. M. (1972, January). *Multimodel techniques and flooding.* Paper presented at the meeting of the Ontario Psychiatric Association Academic Meeting, Toronto.
16. Smith, M. L., Glass, G. V., & Miller, T. L. (1980). *The benefits of psychotherapy.* Baltimore: Johns Hopkins University Press.
17. Locke, H. J., & Wallace, K. (1959). Short marital adjustments and prediction tests. *Marriage and Family Living, 21,* 251–255.
18. Weiss, R. L. (1975). *Spouse observation checklist.* Unpublished Manuscript. University of Oregon.
19. Hops, H., Patterson, G., & Weiss, R. (1971). *Marital interaction coding system.* Unpublished Manuscript. University of Oregon.
20. MacIntosh, D. M. (1975). A comparison of effects of structural, nonshortened training for marital couples. Doctoral Dissertation, North Texas State University. *Dissertation Abstracts International, 36,* 2636–2637A.
21. Venema, H. B. (1975). *Marriage enrichment.* Unpublished doctoral dissertation. Fuller Theological Seminar.
22. Crowe, M. (1978). Conjoint marital therapy: A controlled outcome study. *Psychological Medicine, 8*(4):623–636.
23. Jacobson, N., & Martin, B. (1976). Behavioral marriage therapy: Current status. *Psychological Bulletin, 83,* 540–556.
24. Rosenbluth, M., & Cameron, P. M. (1981). Assessment, commitment and motivation in marital therapy. *Canadian Journal of Psychiatry, 26*(4):151–154.
25. Beck, D., & Jones, M. (1973). *Progress on family problems.* New York: Family Services Association of America.
26. Hartmann, L. (1983). Effects of sex and marital therapy on sexual interaction and marital happiness. *Journal of Sex and Marital Therapy, 9*(2):137–151.
27. Mendonca, J., Lumley, P., & Hunt, A. (1982). Brief marital therapy outcome personality correlates. *Canadian Journal of Psychiatry, 27*(4):291–295.
28. Freeman, S. J., Levens, E. J., & McCulloch, D. J. (1969). Factors

associated with success or failure in marital counselling. *Family Coordinator, 18,* 125-128.
29. Wattie, B. (1973). Evaluating short term case work. *Social Casework, 54,* 609-616.
30. Bowen, M. (1961). The family as the unit of study and treatment. *American Journal of Orthopsychiatry, 31,* 40-60.
31. Slipp, S., & Kressel, K. (1974). Factors associated with engagement in family therapy. *Family Process, 13,* 413-427.
32. Kressel, K., & Slipp, S. (1975). Perceptions of marriage related to engagement in conjoint therapy. *Journal of Marriage and Family Counselling, 1,* 367-377.
33. Santa-Barbara, J., & Epstein, N. (1974). Conflict behavior in clinical families. *Behavioural Sciences, 19,* 100-110.
34. Gurman, A. S. (1974). Attitude change in marital therapy. *Journal of Family Counselling, 2,* 50-54.
35. Griffin, R. W. (1967). Change in perception of marital relationships as related to marriage counselling. *Dissertation Abstracts International, 27,* 39-56A.
36. Santa-Barbara, J., Woodward, C., et al. (1975). *Relationship between therapist characteristics and outcome variable.* Paper presented at Canadian Psychiatric Association, Banff.
37. Rice, D. G., et al. (1972). Therapist experience and style as factors in co-therapy. *Family Process, 11,* 1-12.
38. Woodward, C., Santa-Barbara, J., et al. (1972, April). *Client and therapist characteristics related to family therapy outcome.* Paper presented at the meeting of the American Orthopsychiatry Association, New York.
39. Hollis, F. (1968). Continuance and discontinuance in marital counselling. *Social Casework, 49,* 167-174.
40. Guttman, H., Sigal, J., Epstein, N., & Postner, R. (1971). Process and outcome in conjoint family therapy. *Family Process, 10,* 451-473.
41. Alexander, J., et al. (1976). Systems—Behavioral intervention with families. *Journal of Consulting and Clinical Psychology, 44,* 656-664.
42. Reid, W. J., & Shyne, A. W. (1969). Brief and extended casework. New York: Columbia University Press.
43. Berman, E. M., & Lief, H. I. (1975). Marital therapy from a psychiatric perspective: An overview. *American Journal of Psychiatry, 132*(6):583-592.
44. Karasu, T. (1979). Psychotherapy of medically ill. *American Journal of Psychiatry, 136,* 1-11.
45. Adsett, A., & Bruhn, J. (1968). Short-term group psychotherapy for post myocardial infarction patients and their wives. *Canadian Medical Journal, 99,* 577-584.

46. Gruen, W. (1975). Effects of brief psychotherapy during hospitalization and recovery of heart attacks. *Journal of Consultant Clinical Psychology, 43,* 233.
47. Christensen, D. N. (1983). Post mastectomy counselling: An outcome study. *Journal of Sex and Marital Therapy, 9*(4):266–275.
48. Michels, R., et al. (1984). A debate on DSM-III. *American Journal of Psychiatry, 141*(4):539–553.
49. Livesley, W. J. (1984, October). *Criteria for diagnosis of personality disorder.* Paper presented at the meeting of the Canadian Psychiatric Association, Banff.
50. Shaefer, M. T., & Olsen, D. H. (1981). Assessing intimacy: The pair inventory. *Journal of Marital and Family Therapy,* 47–60.
51. Waring, E. M., et al. (1981). Dimensions of intimacy in marriage. *The Journal of Psychiatry, 44*(2)169–175.
52. Group for the Advancement of Psychiatry (GAP). (1975). *Families in Conflict.* New York: Science House.
53. Waskow, I., & Parloff, M. B. (Eds.). (1975). *Psychotherapy change measures.* Rockville, MD: National Institute of Mental Health.
54. Gurland, B., Yorkston, N. J., Stone, A. R., Frank, J. D., & Fleiss, J. L. (1972, August). The structured and scaled interview to assess maladjustment (SSIAM). I. Description, rationale, and development. *Archives of General Psychiatry, 27,* 259–264.
55. Malan, D. (1976). *The Frontier of brief psychotherapy.* New York: Plenum.
56. Battle, C., Imber, S., & Frank, J. (1966). Target complaints and criteria of improvement. *20,* 184–192.
57. Kiresuk, T., & Shurman, R. (1968). Goal attainment sealing. *Community Mental Health Journal, 4,* 443–453.
58. Candy, J., Marks, I., Malan, D., et al. (1972, November). Psychotherapy outcome research—A feasibility pilot study. *Psychological Medicine.*
59. Gale, A. (1979). Problems of outcome research in family therapy. In S. Walroad-Skinner (Ed.), *Family and Marital Psychotherapy.* London: Routledge & Kegan Paul.
60. Frude, N. (1980). Methodological problems in evolution of family therapy. *Journal of Family Therapy, 2,* 29–44.
61. Lask, B. (1980). Evaluation—Why and how (a guide for clinicians). *Journal of Family Therapy, 2,* 199–210.
62. Rakoff, V., Sigal, J., & Epstein, N. (1975). Predictions of therapeutic process and progress in conjoint family therapy. *General Psychiatry, 32,* 1013.
63. Marks, I. (1978). Behavioral psychotherapy of adult neurosis. In H. Bergin & S. Garfield (Eds.), *Handbook of Psychotherapy and Behavioral Change* (2nd ed.). New York: John Wiley & Sons.

DISCUSSION

Paul G. R. Patterson, M.D.
(University of Western Ontario, Victoria Hospital, London)

I was delighted to be asked to discuss Dr. Cameron's paper because as a child psychiatrist, I am rather concerned about the environment to which children that I see are exposed. An environmental structural model indicates in essence that if the marital union can operate as a self-contained system, containing within itself all the necessary satisfactions and frustrations and object relations of the married pair on one side of the strong generational boundary, then on the other side of the generational boundary the children can be relatively free to grow and develop into healthy, independent, and relatively self-satisfying human beings. If, however, the marital couple cannot contain these things within their marriage but need to breach the generational boundary in order to complete either the individual or the marital systems, then to the degree that this generational boundary has to be breached, the children will be blocked in their development and will present problems. Indeed, as Dr. Cameron has indicated in the beginning of his paper, marital satisfaction is crucial to the quality of life to prevent mental stress and disorder and to ensure healthy psychological and social development. The quality of marital satisfaction affects many more people than the marital couple themselves. It is therefore of paramount importance to know whether a faulty or dysfunctional marital system presents with distress in either of the marital partners or with distress in the children and whether it can be changed by means of therapeutic intervention to become more functional and more satisfying.

In general, scientific research tends to start with some form of inductive method, that is, someone starts with the problem and finds some sort of intervention and then sees whether one of a variety of outcome measures indicates that changes have occurred. Eventually at some point, some general principles are induced from various studies, for example, the fact that certain types of marital therapy for certain types of problems can be effective, and at this point the second or deductive phase of the cycle can begin. We start with the inductive phase and then move to the deductive phase, in which someone comes along, sums up the general principles for us and deduces some specific conclusions from them. After that, and only after that, can the second cycle begin with another inductive phase. This first set of conclusions can be used to design much more specific and refined questions. This first phase of the second cycle then inductively begins to generate a second series of general principles that can be much more specific and much more accurate.

In the area of marital therapy, we are rapidly reaching the end of the first phase of the first cycle—the inductive phase. What Dr. Cameron does is to clarify the principles induced from this first phase; he then takes us through the second phase of the first cycle by deducing for us from this first set of general principles the questions and tools whereby the second and much more specific cycle begins. In other words, what Dr. Cameron has essentially done is to review the state of the art and then has led us gently through the second phase of the first cycle to provide us with all that we need to begin the second cycle. This means we begin to answer the question, "What specific therapy applied to which specific individual's problems and in which specific time by what specific therapist will produce what specific changes?"

I would like to address some specific issues. For instance, in knowing that 30 percent of couples in groups spontaneously improve, what we are not able to do yet at this point in time is to predict which sets of couples those will be. So that is one of the questions to which we have to address ourselves. Knowing that there is a five to 10 percent deterioration rate not only tells us that the procedure is not without some risks but also tells us again that we have to try and develop some way of predicting which five to 10 percent—this is the second question that has to be addressed. Again, as Dr. Cameron pointed out, in many of these situations the question is not which type of therapy works best, but is rather by what criteria can we tell which therapy works best for whom. However, having provided the issues that we need to address, Dr. Cameron was unable at this point in our progress to provide us with any specific recommendations or solutions to these problems, although he coherently outlined both the issues and some of the pitfalls. In the final part of his paper, Dr. Cameron led us quite clearly to the point which I am defining as the end of the first cycle. In essence, he pointed out that we now have sufficient evidence to conclude marital therapy can be effective, that some couples are likely to be helped by any varieties of marital therapy that are available. Some couples are more likely to be helped by one particular variety of marital therapy while other couples would be more likely to be helped by another variety, and still others will need a combination of multiple therapeutic modalities to fully treat their symptoms. Furthermore, Dr. Cameron points out that different types of research designs may be necessary to answer these questions, and that different types of studies can shed light on different aspects of each issue. Finally, Dr. Cameron makes a plea for more eclecticism and collaboration in both formulation of goals and the selection of treatment modalities for the range of distressed marital couples who seek our services and our help.

To summarize, I would suggest to you that the conclusion to be drawn from Dr. Cameron's review of the current state of the art of marital therapy is inescapable. We have arrived at the end of the first cycle of research in this area, and it is high time that we got together to begin the second cycle and to address the question which I cited to you earlier, that is, "What specific therapy will prove most effective for which specific subpopulation of individuals, over what specific period of time, by what specific therapeutic style, to effect which of the number of possible therapeutic goals?" In view of this and in view of the conceptual methodological question raised by Dr. Cameron, these issues must be addressed before this second cycle may productively begin. There is a need to establish priorities, to set up research questions and research directions. It would be helpful to have a common classification system and standardized research design outcome measures that would allow cross-comparison among the studies that need to be done.

In conclusion, I would like to thank Dr. Cameron for providing for the future development of what promises to be a very exciting phase of research in the field of marital therapy. Thank you.

Question: Dr. Cameron, would you like to comment on Dr. Patterson's discussion?

Dr. Cameron: There is an awful lot of data in the literature and it is difficult to know what to pick out in a half an hour. I think that Dr. Patterson has made an important conceptual view of where the state of the literature is, and I fully agree that one follow-up that would be admirable from the viewpoint of this meeting would be for some of us to get together and produce collaborative work. I think this would be extremely helpful. For example, if one reads the literature originating in the United States, one sees that groups there have considerable difficulty collaborating because individuals favor one technique or one set of measurements and on both of those counts if you cannot come to some agreement then it is very difficult for one group of people to know what another group should do. In this country in other areas of psychiatry we have been able to do some good collaborative work because we often are less polarized. If you would like to get together and try to design a specific study using similar populations in different centers, I think that would be by itself very useful.

Dr. Patterson: One of the problems that I find as a clinician and teacher in this area is that I constantly supervise students, trying to help them to recognize the complexity of relationships at all levels, and yet the methodologist coming from another perspective has the opposite task of trying to simplify and categorize data. I wonder if it is really possible for a clinician or teacher to simultaneously perform the research *and* come up with the appropriate methodology for evaluating the type of therapy chosen. Instead, what happens to a lot of us is we start to get defensive as soon as we start reading the research literature and I do not think this should happen. I question whether it is possible for clinicians and teachers to do appropriate research in this area. My objection to the McMaster School of Family Functioning is they could not make up their mind whether this was a way of teaching family therapy or a research instrument for rating family therapy treatment.

Dr. Cameron: I agree with that. I think that we can both influence each other to mutual advantage. I do not like the split quite as much as you stated.

Dr. Patterson: Neither do I in the sense that I am damned if I want a researcher developing the questions unaided and developing the methodology unaided and interpreting his conclusions unaided. On the other hand, a researcher would be a damn fool to let me go off in my heavy clinician's manner and design a study that would end up by proving absolutely nothing. The question that you are raising though is whether clinicians themselves should do the research or whether they should collaborate together.

Dr. Waring: In attempting to answer these questions, one of the dramatic things that has happened in the last

10 years is that the technology of measurement has changed. So I think it is now possible for clinicians and marital therapists to do very useful practice audits that come very close to good outcome studies by simply utilizing the technology of measurement as well as doing the usual things, such as asking your patients whether they feel they have been helped, whether they feel better, worse, or whatever, and making your independent judgments. You can use some valid, reliable instruments independently, and oddly enough since we have been doing that for a while, one thing that strikes me is how much the couples like to do these things before and after therapy. They really enjoy the procedure of filling out self-report questionnaires and getting feedback about it as part of the assessment process, and oddly enough they really enjoy being seen by raters. Not all clinicians can do that obviously—have somebody else see them to do an assessment. Couples seem to enjoy the whole process of being objectively evaluated and then getting feedback at the end as to how they did. One of the issues that Paul raises is when you get this multiple feedback on your practice, you learn very quickly which patients are doing well and which are not, which you are effective with and which you are not. So it is not as hard to do as it was a decade ago.

Question: One of the problems that I see is that almost all therapies seem to have a 70 percent success rate as a cutoff point. We had a visitor from Milwaukee from a strategic family therapy center last week, who said very proudly that they had a 70 percent success rate. But for me the point is, What do you do with the other 30 percent? I have not seen any studies that proceed to examine that 30 percent in any great detail and to assign these individuals to different types of therapies and to try to find out the characteristics of these people. I agree with you that a collaborative study should be done involving various centers that use a defined treatment modality, and that then would pool their 30 percent treatment failures and redistribute these individuals among different treatment modalities. I think this is what you would call the second stage of research. That is where we have to go. It has been pretty satisfactorily demonstrated that we have achieved a 70 percent success rate.

Chapter 7

TRANSFERENCE AND COUNTER-TRANSFERENCE IN MARITAL THERAPY

Herta A. Guttman

Historically, family therapy theorists have emphasized transactional rules in the here and now and have tended to deny or downplay the importance of the fantasies and projected images from the past that underlie transference and countertransference reactions.[1-4] Nevertheless, it has long been recognized that a therapeutic situation involving the spouse of a patient who is in individual therapy can be a powerful stimulus for these phenomena to arise. Giovacchini used the term *triangular transference* to denote the archaic conflicts that are expressed in the patient's dreams, fantasies, and acting out, in reaction to the contact between his or her spouse and the therapist.[5] Greene and Solomon, in discussing the repercussions of concurrent but separate therapy of husband and wife, coined the phrase *triangular transference transactions* to describe the emergence of transference reactions involving both the spouse and the therapist.[6] Indeed, Dicks' classical observation of married couples emphasized the importance in the marital relationship of projective identification and reciprocal unconscious role expectations deriving from the spouses' families of origin.[7] However, Dicks did not include the therapist as an object of transference nor did he consider his or her countertransference feelings.

In family therapy, the realistic aspects of the therapy situation are assumed to be predominant, the therapist being viewed as an objective agent of change who is not endowed with any unrealistic expectations by the clients.[3] Similarly, the therapist's reciprocal feelings and fantasies are minimized. The therapeutic alliance is therefore considered to be much more significant than transference or countertransference and has been described as *joining* the family.[10]

Family therapists have certainly recognized the enormous importance of triangular relationships and triadic situations in family life and have repeatedly demonstrated that triadic experiences can be a powerful source of growth,[8] a refuge from the potential suffocation of a dyadic relationship,[9] or a source of inappropriate cross-generational coalitions.[10] In later life, such relationships continue to be very powerful, because of early formative experiences which have usually involved a triad or a triangle. The triadic situation of couple therapy, therefore, is especially prone to evoke thoughts, feelings, fantasies, and behavior patterns that are related to each spouse's personal history and to his or her position and affective experiences in the family of origin.[11-13] For the same reason, couple therapy can evoke strong feelings in the therapist. To be effective, he or she must learn to recognize, understand, and cope with these feelings.

In couple therapy, triadic situations occur in the context of a deeply affective relationship in which sex and sexual passion usually have played a central role. It is therefore most convenient to consider transference processes as being nonsexualized or sexualized.

SPOUSES' NONSEXUALIZED TRANSFERENCE REACTIONS

Symmetrical Reactions

In this situation, the therapist is perceived either as a nurturant or a withholding parent by one or both members of the couple, who assume the role of siblings with respect to each other and of children with respect to the therapist.

Competition. The most frequent type of sibling response is negative and symmetrical: that is, to be jealous of or competitive with the spouse, and to vie for the therapist's attention and preference. This is overtly expressed in the desire to have the therapist judge which of them is "right." Although this wish is almost always expressed to some extent—particularly at the beginning of therapy—it can be prolonged and exaggerated with certain couples.

Union. A rarer occurrence is a symmetrical situation in which both members of the couple see the therapist as a bad, withholding parent and unite against him or her. In one such case, both spouses were troubled people with personality disorders which could be described as borderline.[14] In spite of being highly intelligent and gifted, they found it extremely difficult to organize their lives and to take responsibility for their little daughter. Whenever they were confronted with the demands of sober reality, they would fight, argue, blame one another and often would act out sexually against each other. Once in therapy, these disagreements became rarer: This couple seemed to have found a kind of togetherness by uniting through playfulness, flirtation, and secrets which excluded the therapist, whom they obviously perceived as a bad, judgmental parent. The tendency to object splitting so common in borderline personalities found its expression in a solution that united them against the therapist and permitted them to function more harmoniously with each other. Prior to therapy, they had essentially tried the same solution through "swinging" with another couple and then uniting with each other against this other, "bad" couple. The stability of their marriage therefore depended on the presence of a third party who could serve as a bad object. Their need for the continued presence of a bad object resulted in a therapeutic stalemate. Either the therapist had to continue serving this function indefinitely or therapy had to be terminated.

Asymmetrical Reactions

The spouse as caretaker. In asymmetrical relationships, one spouse may experience deep longing for parental sustenance and protection, which it is the other spouse's function to provide. Such marriages have been called "caretaker" or "doll's house" marriages.[15] If, in therapy, the "caretaken" spouse turns to the therapist for nurturance, the "caretaker" spouse may feel threatened by loss of this role and can sabotage treatment. In one instance, a recently married couple came to therapy, on the recommendation of a neurologist who could find nothing to explain why the wife—a longtime sufferer from seizure disorder—had had an increasing number of uncontrollable seizures since the marriage. The husband came with a diary, detailing the chronology and consequences of each convulsion. He had clearly hoped to take such good care of his wife that he would "cure" her epilepsy after their marriage. As the therapist began encouraging the wife to express herself, it emerged that she was unhappy with her husband's rather egocentric behavior in other areas of their life. In response, the husband became increasingly vocal, reiterating that the main problem was the wife's epilepsy and urging the therapist to make renewed contact with the referring neurologist.

The spouse as auxiliary therapist. Alternatively, the "caretaker" partner may try to retain his or her role by joining rather than competing with the therapist in caring for his "sick" spouse. In my experience this reaction is especially common in spouses who have had the role of a parental child in their families of origin and have learned to deal with their own need for nurturance by identification with a younger needy sibling. In one such case, a middle-aged professional man developed a major depression, necessitating many changes of medication before an effective one was found. His wife, who had always resented but tolerated his close relationship with a demanding mother, became more openly contemptuous of his anxious dependence. She, herself, had been the devoted oldest daughter in a large immigrant family. Marrying a successful professional man had probably counterbalanced her anger at his dependence on his mother. After he became ill, however, she had to contend not only with an overbearing mother-in-law but also with an "expert" therapist. Nevertheless, she only complained about her husband's tie to his *mother*, joining the therapist in monitoring her husband's progress and his response to the medication.

Therapeutic Strategies

Fairness. The therapist must be aware of his/her power to stimulate primitive, regressive wishes in each spouse, and must be prepared to make interventions that take such transference reactions into account. In most cases, the therapeutic alliance is sufficiently strong to permit useful therapy. Simply by being fair and allotting adequate attention to each person in turn, the therapist can limit the sibling rivalry that is aroused, because much of it results from the competitive anxiety of a triadic situation.

However, in some cases it is necessary either to investigate and interpret the situation further or to find some other way of neutralizing a triangular transference situation that is potentially destructive.

Psychogenetic reconstruction with interpretation. Tracing and connecting the feelings and behavior of each person back to that person's experience in his or her family of origin has value because it fosters greater mutual empathy and allows the couple to overcome barriers to their relationship that arise out of their past experience. For instance, early in therapy a husband felt that the therapist was always siding with his wife because she did not actively take part in arguments between them, preferring to make reflective and introspective remarks to both of them. It emerged that he had always felt that his father respected and loved his only sibling, a brother, more than himself. His wife had felt similarly criticized and disfavored by her mother, in contrast to her younger brother. Whereas she relaxed and felt understood simply because she was listened to and not criticized by the female therapist, the husband felt himself attacked as he had been in his family of origin. The therapist's parental role vis-à-vis each spouse was in conflict with the image the other spouse developed. Reconstruction of this experience permitted treatment to continue, whereas it may otherwise have resulted in a stalemate. It also gave the couple greater empathy for one another in other situations.

Using the transference. It is sometimes more advantageous temporarily to use rather than to interpret the reactions aroused by the therapeutic situation. A middle-aged couple came for therapy because of a crisis in their relationship, which had been triggered by the fact that the wife had for several months submerged herself in decorating a new apartment for their 27-year-old daughter who—according to the husband—had always been "spoiled rotten" by his wife. He reacted very angrily to his wife's preoccupation and threatened to divorce her if she did not change. The husband also reported feeling depressed, not concentrating well at work, and not getting along well with a new boss.

The husband immediately bonded with the therapist. It became clear that she represented what he had always wished for: an involved nurturant mother, unlike his own divorced mother who had viewed him primarily as a support in caring for his older, manic-depressive brother who claimed all her attention. Clearly, his wife's involvement with their daughter had revived much of his hurt and resentment toward his mother.

By initially giving the husband a lot of attention, the therapist fostered his positive transference to alleviate his depression and allow him to regain functioning. She kept the wife as an ally by temporarily conferring on the husband the role of a sick, depressed person and enlisting the wife's cooperation in caring for him. Within three sessions the husband regained some self-esteem, his mood improved, and the therapist could then be more impartial and begin helping the couple with their long-standing problems.

As with the "splitting" couple described earlier, however, these triangular transference situations sometimes create a stalemate because one or both partners cannot transcend the transference with an observing ego. The therapist may then choose to continue serving indefinitely as a stabilizing influence in an explosive, regressive situation, accept failure, or find a way of uniting the couple by serving as a permanently bad object.

SPOUSES' SEXUALIZED TRANSFERENCE REACTIONS

In this situation, one member of the couple is sexually attracted to the therapist and the other becomes sexually jealous and possessive. This situation can quickly become explosive or can lead to a therapeutic impasse. It is particularly problematic when both therapist and couple are young and attractive and the therapist lacks experience.

Heterosexual Triangulation

Interpretation. In such situations, feelings that are being aroused by the triadic situation should be interpreted as soon as they are relatively clear. In one case, the husband complimented a female therapist on her attractive dress. As soon as she had an opportunity in that interview, the therapist asked the wife how she felt about her husband's remark. This led to a discussion of the partners' feelings, attitudes, and doubts regarding marital infidelity, which—as it turned out—had been a issue for them for many years. This intervention ensured that they continued coming to therapy and also opened up an important area for therapeutic intervention.

Challenge. If this situation is not addressed, therapy can be unproductive. In a typical case, a young, attractive, and rather histrionic wife insisted on couple therapy because she felt her husband was cold, undemonstrative, and domineering and because she wanted to start a family but was dubious about the strength of their relationship. She soon began turning to the young male therapist for advice and comfort and as arbiter between herself and her husband. The husband, an obsessional young man who was not at all in touch with his feelings, turned the therapy into a struggle between the therapist and himself by being consistently late for appointments and smilingly disqualifying the importance of his lateness. The therapist became increasingly frustrated and angry while feeling totally powerless. Soon, the wife became pregnant, the couple said their relationship had improved, and they withdrew from therapy. Although he was aware that this sexualized triangle was impeding therapy, the therapist had not been able to find a way of dealing with the situation, perhaps because the wife was an attractive young woman whose dependence appealed to him, or perhaps because he feared his strong feelings of anger toward the husband.

Reconciliation. Sometimes, rather than interpreting it, the therapist can use the sexualized transference situation to reconcile two warring partners. Minuchin describes such a situation in which, instead of acknowledging it, he dealt with the wife's sexualized transference to him by mildly insulting her, thereby forcing her to ally with her husband against him.[10]

Homosexual triangulation. A rarer occurrence, and one which is less well recognized, is a homosexual triangular transference situation, in which the same-sex partner is attracted to the therapist and the opposite-sex partner reacts with possessiveness and hostility. Unless the therapist is aware of this possibility, because its homoerotic elements can be well disguised, such behavior can appear to be the nonsexualized competition for nurturance, which has already been described.

Both types of sexualized transference feelings often emerge after a switch from individual to couple therapy. Either the former individual patient or the spouse demonstrates feelings of sexual rivalry toward the therapist or toward the spouse. In one case, a homosexual transference rivalry developed after a female therapist switched from individual therapy with the wife to couple therapy. The wife was previously aware of having lesbian feelings.

During individual therapy it became clear that when she was feeling insecure she would turn to another, stronger woman for support and would then develop homosexual desires that frightened her. These had abated in individual therapy. During the early couple sessions the wife reported jealous, possessive feelings about the therapist and described thinly disguised homoerotic dreams. The therapist first ignored the homoerotic aspects of this transference, simply interpreting the patient's anger that she must now share her therapist with her husband. Later, as the therapeutic alliance with the husband become stronger, the wife's homosexual conflicts were also openly discussed.

Methods of Intervening

It is not always necessary to appeal to insight in order to deal with the transferential component of marital interaction. Some therapists try to modify communication patterns or assign tasks, in an effort to alter various stereotyped patterns of behavior or perception. These techniques can directly induce new behavior or they may indirectly alter it, by making it impossible simultaneously to comply with the task and to continue in the same way as before.

Some therapists use techniques derived from psychodrama and Gestalt therapy, such as doubling, role reversal or sculpting. *Doubling* is useful when one spouse cannot directly confront the other. The therapist can communicate this person's putative feelings on his or her behalf, at the same time serving a protective role by deliberately triangulating the interaction, so that either spouse can reject the feelings if they are too dangerous and can insist they were invented by the therapist.

Role reversal is an important technique for heightening empathy and can be useful with narcissistic partners who are not easily capable of seeing things from another's point of view. Role reversal also permits one spouse to show the other how he or she would like to communicate. In the process, the therapist's salience can be reduced to that of a go-between rather than a principal.[16]

Sculpting techniques[17] are appropriate for spouses who "bury" each other and the therapist under a barrage of words. The silence of sculpting provides a medium for affect, empathy, and insight to emerge.

It is important to understand that any one of these interventions can in turn induce transference reactions. For instance, the therapist can be viewed as a primitive "magical" parent, an intrusive punitive parent, or a demanding perfectionistic parent. His or her physical closeness during sculpting can evoke a wish for even greater intimacy or an intolerable fear of suffocation. Such reactions require immediate explication, lest they interfere with the therapeutic movement that can be gained from using these techniques.

THE THERAPIST'S COUNTERTRANSFERENCE REACTIONS

Whereas the experience of being in a triangular situation is fundamental to our earliest memories of family life, it is—paradoxically—one of the most difficult to manage successfully, as witnessed by the saying, "Two's company, three's a crowd." Triads too often become coalitions of two against one, fusion of two or three members into pseudomutuality, or distantiation between members in order to avoid fusion.

The triangular situation of couple therapy arouses affects, fantasies, and memories in the therapist as well as in the couple. These countertransferential experiences can be a help or a hindrance to the therapist, according to the way in which they are used. Most often, in marital therapy, therapists find themselves cast in the role of a parent or a child-sibling, each of which gives rise to characteristic countertransference problems.

Parental Countertransference

Being cast in the role of a parent can reactivate a strong oedipal conflict. The therapist may seductively join one partner to the exclusion or humiliation of the other. Particularly for younger therapists, it can be most difficult to recognize and tolerate any sort of parentification, especially by people to whom he or she is sexually attracted or by people who are considerably older.

"Child" Countertransference

On the other hand, the therapist who has strong "child" needs may misperceive the parentified role that is being thrust on him or her as a sibling role. If he or she always wanted to be favored vis-à-vis a sibling, the therapist may unconsciously foster and enjoy a coalition with the spouse who represents a parent in his or her eyes, leaving the other spouse out of the picture.

When one is treating a couple who are always arguing and fighting, this experience can arouse feelings of being a helpless, overwhelmed child caught between warring parents. This situation can provoke silence, inactivity, or withdrawal on the part of the therapist.

Therapeutic Strategies

By some process which is subjective and not entirely explicable, therapists often manage appropriate therapeutic behavior as long as they are aware of their feelings. If they are unaware of their reactions to the couple, their inappropriate responses can range from being chronically late for sessions to constantly putting the same spouse (the rival) on the spot, from finding a way of prematurely terminating the case to ignoring blatantly provocative statements or behavior on the part of the couple.

Various types of appropriate therapeutic behavior have been described in this paper. They include conscious fairness in allotting one's attention; interventions that deliberately disclaim the responsibility of being a judge; interpretations that explore the partners' unconscious expectations that the therapist will be an ally, a rival, or a parent; interpretations connecting present behavior to past conditioning; or careful use of the transference to further a particular goal. The therapist may even reveal countertransference feelings in a therapeutic way; for example, "The two of you are making me feel like a parent with two small kids. Who should get my attention first?"

Sometimes even the most experienced therapist can profit from a consultation that clarifies countertransference distortions that are impeding therapy. A particularly powerful modality of consultation is that of strategic family therapy, in which the therapist and the couple are viewed by a group through a one-way mirror, with the group intervening with a message or a prescription that is usually couched in the manner of the "Greek chorus."[18,19] Such consultations can be for one session only, or—with particularly difficult and rigid couple systems in which the therapist has become a stabilizer rather than an agent of change—they can become the most viable therapeutic modality. The technique of offering such consultation is still in its early stages. It offers the advantage of powerfully detriangulating the therapeutic system by offering a "quadrad" instead of a triad, thereby providing the therapist with an ally who can usefully extricate him or her from nonproductive countertransference reactions. Moreover, the group can help the therapist by provoking a couple in chronic conflict to unite with him or her against them,[18] thereby providing a basis for marital harmony.

In summary, whatever the modality or process of coming to terms with countertransference, to the extent that the therapist recognizes, uses, or seeks help in neutralizing the less conscious components of his or her reactions, he or she will have mobilized one of the important aspects of being therapeutic.

THEORETICAL IMPLICATIONS

It is not a new assumption that the marital relationship rests, at least in part, on expectations and perceptions that have been transferred from each partner's earlier significant life experiences.[7,11,12,20] To the extent that such "transferences" are gratified or corroborated, the marital relationship may be satisfactory.

However, two less satisfactory eventualities can occur in marriage: (1) one or several key expectations are sorely disappointed, the partner even turning out to be the reverse of what he or she appeared to be during the courtship;[7] (2) a life crisis of some sort forces a shift in the marital equilibrium, so that the previous "transference" need is no longer gratified. An example of the first eventuality would be one of a woman who marries a man because he is "the life of the party," gratifying her repressed exhibitionistic needs and also being the opposite of her harsh, puritanical father. However, she eventually becomes embarrassed by her husband's expansive clowning and begins to criticize him for just the quality she previously appreciated. An example of the second eventuality is evident with the "swinging" couple described earlier in this paper. Their contract to be playmates, united against disapproving parents, was successful until they themselves became parents and could no longer sustain these roles.

Our terminology for conceptualizing both these eventualities as they occur in the marital relationship is still somewhat vague and not sufficiently comprehensive. Projective identification, as described by Dicks,[7] is not identical with transference, insofar as the term only refers to the projection of "disavowed and disallowed" parts of the self onto the marital partner. These are not necessarily synonymous with unconsciously introjected and repressed perceptions or expectations of a significant other that are then projected onto the spouse. They are not at all synonymous with the unconscious perception or memory of a *relationship* that has been previously observed or experienced and is transferred to the marital relationship. For these reasons, the concept of transference adds another dimension to Dicks' paradigm, because it implies a *relationship* with another person.

Should one use the terms "transference" and "countertransference" to designate such phenomena? Although the term "transference" is often restricted to the process whereby the patient transfers exclusively to the therapist a complex of thoughts, feelings, and fantasies about a person who was important in his or her past life, Freud emphasized that transference is a universal phenomenon and that every meaningful relationship contains transference elements.[21] Brenner is of the opinion that all relationships contain transference elements and emphasizes that it is the therapist's neutral, analytic response and not the transference itself that makes the therapist-patient relationship different from others.[22] However, it may in fact be preferable to distinguish between the therapist-patient and real-life relationships by using a different term, such as "parataxic distortion" as proposed by Sullivan,[23] to characterize nonpatient-therapist experiences.

The occurrence of these transference-like processes raises the further question of identifying the curative factor in marital therapy. In individual psychoanalytic therapy cure is attributed to successful analysis of the transference relationship. This is because it is assumed to reproduce the reality-based experiences that have given the patient success and difficulty, pleasure and pain in real life. In the absence of a real relationship in the therapy situation, the transference is the patient's and the analyst's window on the patient's real world. Furthermore, the basic unreality of the therapist-patient relationship weakens resistance and gives transference interpretations a particular force. In the face of the therapist's neutral behavior, the irrationality of the patient's reactions and distortions become all the more obvious.[22]

None of this supposedly occurs in marital therapy, because the therapist is more active, the marital partner is real. Whatever transference exists within the marital relationship is thought to be more difficult to "dislodge," because, unlike the neutral therapist in individual therapy, the spouse constantly reinforces these distorted perceptions by his or her behavior. Therefore, the therapist's transference interpretations do not have the same impact, being obscured by the real behavior of the partner. Moreover, some therapists fear that, if it is successful, marital therapy that focuses on transference phenomena between the partners has the unfortunate consequence of encouraging them to become objective, empathic therapeutic agents for one another, thereby devitalizing a relationship that should be spontaneous and passionate.[24]

This is not a valid argument. As this paper has demonstrated, a prior transference-like relationship between the spouses is a "given" in all marriages. To this is added the particular triadic situation of conjoint couple therapy, involving parataxic distortions between the partners and the therapist. Both the dyadic and triadic aspects of this situation rapidly heighten certain marital conflicts, permitting the therapist to gain insight into their significance. This probably also hastens the interpretation and the working through of feelings and attitudes toward the spouse because the other person is present in the session, rather than being outside the therapy situation, as in the cases described by Giovacchini and by Greene and Solomon.[5,6] The phenomenon of temporarily decreased spontaneity and a tendency to become overinvolved with oneself occurs in individual therapy as well as in marital therapy. In both cases, this may result in a temporary cooling of conjugal spontaneity and passion, but it is not a lasting problem in most marital relationships.

Another view of the curative ingredient in marital therapy holds that the mutual and collusive transferences that have been described are equivalent to resistances in individual therapy, so that the real work of marital therapy can only occur once these transferences are removed. This is in contrast to individual therapy, where the real work of the treatment is said to be the analysis and the removal of the transference, including the resistances connected with it.[25,26] In my view, the attenuation of resistance through transference interpretations does not alone lead to change, either in individual or in couple therapy. Rather, it is the working-through process, which involves not only insight into past patterns and their unconscious determinants but also actively seeking new responses, interactions, and attitudes. For therapy of any kind to be deemed successful, the individual or the couple must not only modify their perceptions or expectations and increase their insight, but must also develop a more satisfying relationship.

In this view, conjoint couple therapy therefore remains within the tradition of individual therapy, with respect to the theory of its effectiveness and the place of transference and of countertransference phenomena in the working-through process. What remains unresolved is a more satisfactory terminology to describe the mechanisms and origins of these phenomena.

REFERENCES

1. Ackerman, N.W. (1962). Family psychotherapy and psychoanalysis: The implications of difference. *Family Process, 1,* 30–43.
2. Haley, J. (1970). Approaches to family therapy. *International Journal of Psychiatry, 9,* 233–242.
3. Epstein, N.B., Sigal, J.J., & Rakoff, V. (1966). Some issues in family therapy. *Laval Medical, 37,* 146–150.

4. Jackson, D.D., & Weakland, J.H. (1961). Conjoint family therapy: Some considerations on theory, technique and results. *Psychiatry, 24,* 30-45.
5. Giovacchini, P.L. (1965). Treatment of marital disharmonies: The classical approach. In B.L. Greene (Ed.), *The psychotherapies of marital disharmony.* New York: The Free Press.
6. Greene, B.L., & Solomon, A.P. (1963). Marital disharmony: Concurrent psychoanalytic therapy of husband and wife by the same psychiatrist—the triangular transference transactions. *American Journal of Psychotherapy, 17,* 443-456.
7. Dicks, H. (1967). *Marital tensions.* New York: Basic Books.
8. Satir, V. (1980, August). Conference '80, Val Morin, Quebec.
9. Anonymous. (1972). Towards the differentiation of a self in one's own family. In J. Framo (Ed.), *Family interaction: A dialogue between family researchers and family therapists,* (pp. 111-173). New York: Springer.
10. Minuchin, S. (1974). *Families and family therapy.* Cambridge, MA: Harvard University Press.
11. Greenspan, S.I., & Mannino, F.V. (1974). A model for brief intervention with couples based on projective identification. *American Journal of Psychiatry, 131,* 1103-1106.
12. Grunebaum, H., & Christ, J. (1968). Interpretation and the task of the therapist with couples and families. *International Journal of Group Psychotherapy, 18,* 495-503.
13. Sager, C.J. (1967). Transference in conjoint treatment of married couples. *Archives of General Psychiatry, 16,* 185-193.
14. Gunderson, J.G., & Singer, M.T. (1975). Defining borderline patients: An overview. *American Journal of Psychiatry, 132,* 1-10.
15. Pittman, F.S., & Flomenhaft, K. (1970). Treating the doll's house marriage. *Family Process, 9,* 143-155.
16. Zuk, G.H. (1966). The "go-between" process in family therapy. *Family Process, 5,* 162-177.
17. Papp, P. (1982). Reciprocal metaphors in a couples group. *Family Process, 21,* 453-468.
18. Papp, P. (1980). The Greek chorus and other techniques of family therapy. *Family Process, 19,* 45-58.
19. Palazzoli-Selvini, M., Boscolo, L., Cecchin, G., & Prata, G. (1980). Hypothesizing–circularity–neutrality: Three guidelines for the conductor of the session. *Family Process, 19,* 3-12.
20. Paul, N. (1967). The role of mourning and empathy in conjoint marital therapy. In G. Zuk & I. Boszormenyi-Nagy (Eds.), *Family therapy and disturbed families* (pp. 186-206). Palo Alto: Science and Behavior Books.

21. Orr, D.W. (1954). Transference and countertransference: A historical survey. *Journal of the American Psychoanalytic Association 2*, 621–669.
22. Brenner, C. (1976). Psychoanalytic technique and psychic conflict. New York: International Universities Press.
23. Mullahy, P. (1970). *Psychoanalysis and interpersonal psychiatry* (pp. 337–339). New York: Science House.
24. Aldous, N.R. (1979). *Discussion of Saul Albert Memorial Lecture: Marriage and marital therapy from an object relations viewpoint.* Paper presented by J. Framo at the Jewish General Hospital, Montreal.
25. Gurman, A.S. (1978). Contemporary marital therapies: A critique and comparative analysis of psychoanalytic, behavioral and systems theory approaches. Transference, its role in conjoint therapy. In T.J. Paolino & B.S. McCrady (Eds.), *Marriage and marital therapy* (pp. 467–472). New York: Brunner/Mazel.
26. Watters, W. (1980). Personal communication.

DISCUSSION

Lila Russell, M.S.W. *(Victoria Hospital, London)*

The reciprocal unconscious role expectations derived from each spouse's family of origin can certainly wreak havoc on the marital relationship. Clifford Sager, in *Marriage Contracts and Couple Therapy,** provides an account of how these hidden forces in intimate relationships can be brought to consciousness. He facilitates the negotiation of new contracts, which are healthier for the couple's survival. It has been said that there are as many theories and therapies for couples in conflict as there are therapists. Many schools, as you point out, minimize the importance of unconscious forces in favor of simply modifying the behavior in the here-and-now. Many family therapy schools do, of course, downplay the power of introjected parental messages and bypass them in therapy. Other therapists

---

* New York: Brunner/Mazel, 1976.

describe these introjections as projections of the identified problem of those marriages that are falling apart. The transference/countertransference phenomena are always partially activated in the therapist's alliance, and it is necessary for the therapist to be aware of them and to actively or intellectually deal with them somehow.

I am not quite sure where we go from there. In my opinion, the working-through process, which involves insight into past patterns and their unconscious, is not always necessary. Often the couple is enabled to modify the perception and their expectations of one another through other models of therapy. For example, Waring described one such method, cognitive family therapy, to deal with some of these phenomena. I wish to emphasize, however, that the therapist's self-awareness is crucial, and this could be defined as the conscious recognition of one's own motivation and feeling, and behavior.

Understanding the self enables the therapists to be sensitive and, hence, to prevent their own anxious feelings from interfering with the assessment and treatment of couples. The therapist's own dynamics may enable the creation of relationships with a varying degree of freedom or inhibit couple responses altogether, because the couple are saying some pretty overwhelming things. For example, our technique may be too intense and frightening, and a young therapist may have to block it. It is important to ensure that these problems and blind spots do not limit professional usefulness.

Countertransference is often a part of the therapeutic process. It is important for the therapist to be aware of this in order to be able to recognize countertransference issues in a variety of ways, which promotes responsible professional attitudes. When the therapist's countertransference is activated, it is important to know where these feelings stem from. In one example, the therapist says to the couple, "The two of you make me feel like a parent with two fighting kids." This is acceptable, and the therapist is absolutely sure that this couple provokes these feelings in all observers and that it is not stemming from the old feelings that the therapist had in his or her family of origin.

It is well known that many go into the helping professions in a search for self-cure. On the whole, these sex therapists are sensitive, warm people who enjoy helping others. They embark upon a vigorous training program and develop a body of knowledge and many skills through their various internships. They are exposed to extensive supervision during training years, in which they are forced to look into their own personality, develop self-awareness, and adopt humanistic attitudes. Through ongoing supervision, consultation, and personal therapy, these therapists are learning to control feelings and the expression of attitudes, which are considered destructive to the therapeutic relationship.

Michael Nichols, in a book called *Family Therapy*,* provides a useful description of the various schools of family therapy that promotes further configuration and use of terms like transference and countertransference. He points out that more and more psychoanalytically trained clinicians are practicing family therapy today, using methods consistent with their training. These practitioners come to work in the same setting and with similar patients as do individual psychoanalytical therapists. They are working largely with verbal, intelligent, middle-class patients who are not seriously disturbed. The method of self-discovery relies heavily on words, and it works best with articulate patients who are motivated to learn about themselves. This, of course, may be out of place for people struggling with a serious type of pathological or situational stress, but for the repressed neurotic these techniques can give new light into their days of anxiety and apathy.

Couples with high anxiety/low motivation, I believe,

---

* New York: Gardner Press, 1984.

do much better with the action-oriented approach—Minuchin's structural or Haley's strategic therapy. Behavior marital therapy works best with couples who want action, who want to be told what to do, and will follow directions. Being able to integrate a variety of therapy models with your own personality works best for those people who have a thorough background of training and supervision in some form of family therapy; I do not really think it matters which form as long as it is thorough, because once you know one thing well, you can then expand and begin to learn to use other models. I do not think periodic attendance at workshops substitutes for an appropriate apprenticeship, but I think workshops are good at enhancing skills of already experienced practitioners. The trend toward conversion is illustrated by Haley's incorporation into his strategic therapy of structural concepts by behaviorists, who are increasingly taking into account the nonobservable experience, such as cognition, affect, attitude, motivation, and by the widespread use of certain techniques developed by the Milan Group, including clarifying communication, reframing, and paradox.

The most useful theories of family functioning treat families as systems, have concepts that describe forces for stability and change, consider the past but concentrate on the present, treat communication as multilevel and complex, recognize the triadic nature of human relationships, remember to consider the context of the nuclear family rather than viewing it as a closed system isolated from its environment, and recognize the critical function of boundaries in protecting the cohesiveness of individuals, couples, and family.

The broad goals of family therapy are to solve presenting problems and to reorganize the family system. Some of the major differences among family therapists on how behavior is changed are focused on the following issues: action or insight, change in session or change at home, duration of treatment, resistance, couple/therapist relationship, and paradox. Even though there is a general consensus about some of the issues, most therapists believe action is primary and insight is useful but secondary. There are divergent opinions on every one of these points. The job of the theoretician is to decode and decipher. It requires the use of ingenuity to discover patterns. The job of the therapist is to cure; it requires theory but also power, perseverance, and caring. Treating couples in conflict is not only based on science or technology, it is also an art carried out in a framework of humanitarian concern. Perhaps this is countertransference, but if it is within the therapist's control and awareness, the therapeutic alliance is then free to focus on providing the couple with support, with respect, and with acceptance.

Dr. Waring: As I understand, in the development of transference in individual therapy, most authors talk initially about a reaction—a conscious emotion that they have towards the therapist. The emotion is quite available to the patient, but people debate this. Then, you get into material about the patient, which is consciously withheld, or you get into disclosure; again, not unconscious material, it is just material that people do not like to reveal, at least initially. The idea was that transference behaviors by the patient with the analyst start to emerge somewhere around six to 10 sessions, become more obvious, and the analyst would identify this pattern as a transference pattern. Perhaps the person was not producing any material or was coming late, and then this would lead to an understanding about unconscious material.

If that is true, then in many of the major short marital therapies, the couple is finished before transference has developed. I would like you to comment on whether or not you think it is true that unconscious transference may not have developed within eight to 10 sessions, whereas it would in longer-term sessions?

The second part of the question is: In the longer-term sessions, does the resolution of transference behavior become part of the therapeutic cure—if you wish, part of the focus rather than the initial problem?

The second question is the reverse. I have been told by many people that they see the brief kinds of marital therapy focusing on communication or skills, as being designed to facilitate positive transference; they have built in positive transference. I wonder if you would comment on this.

Dr. Guttman: I will try. Even 10 sessions, I think, require something like 10 weeks, so that they are brief for us; and we are not talking about people who stop thinking or reacting the minute they leave our office, anymore than we do. I think that we have to situate it in terms of time, that even in 10 weeks you can develop a lot of feelings. I think it is absolutely paramount to distinguish between transference and the therapeutic alliance; whether it is negative or positive is by its very definition conscious. Transference by its very definition, correct me if I am wrong, is not only negative it is also positive because idealization is part of transference, which refers to anything that is unconscious by its very definition. Transference is usually a desire related to fantasies that are self-generated or that are triggered by past unresolved or unfulfilled experiences, or very fulfilling experiences, which one wishes to repeat in the present. Therefore, transference is always used in terms of the negative aspects only, but we should realize that each of these reactions can have a positive or negative effect.

If you trace this historically to Freud, he originally commented on transference as being simply a specific manifestation of a process that occurs between any two people in any situation. Brenner further elaborated that the main difference between the phenomena that occur in analysis and other therapy, and elsewhere, is that the therapist is inactive, the therapist does not respond like a true, live human being to the projections of the patient. However, a therapist has his or her own unconscious expectations and fantasies, and unconsciously motivated behaviors. For example, you have Laing who says that whatever you do, you have done something, which is more important than anything else in your office. Since I come from a department that has a large nucleus of Laing followers, I am quite familiar with all these, but I think you have to distinguish all this from marital and family therapy, which by their very nature are more active. The marital or family therapist is more active, the therapist is "real," and has very vital interactions with the couple or the family. Therefore, the therapist probably discloses more inadvertently, or by the very nature of his or her behavior, and then there is more material for transference expectations and transference reactions to occur.

I would also like to say that I, personally, do not have too much trouble with positive transference or a positive therapeutic alliance in the context of marital or family therapy. I do not think that it has to be analyzed, I do not think it has to be commented on; it is not the same as psychoanalysis. On the contrary, it is the negative aspects that I concentrated on in my paper. I am basically dealing with the ways in which you can deal with negative transference. I am sure that negative transference arises much more quickly in couple and family therapy of any kind than in so-called brief therapy.

Dr. Rosenbluth: We know from the marital therapy literature, and I know from an informal survey I have conducted, that marital therapy lasts different lengths of time—from 10 to 12 sessions to 2 years or longer, by Dr. Martin for some of his cases. Some of us fall in between in terms of an average, and so we are talking about different things. Thus your paper and what it deals with has different implications, I think, for the couple you are working with in 10 sessions, where transference reactions are very important to recognize and to use insofar as they color the development of allies, as you were pointing out. This is very different from more intensive marital therapy, where one might work with a couple for longer than 10 or 12 sessions. I would suggest that if you work with a couple for half a year to two years, transference rather than transference reaction comes more into play. Similarly, countertransference rather than countertransference reactions comes into play; therefore, I think the duration is one thing that has to be kept in mind. The other aspect, which I think is interesting to consider, is that even in 10 sessions of marital therapy there is very strong transference as opposed to transference reaction; it is not from the spouse to the therapist, it is transference that walks through the door. The beauty and interesting thing about marital therapy is that you do not have to sit around and put in your two years with a patient waiting for a transference to develop and work through.

The clinical issues to consider are: when is the identification of the transference to the spouse; what is the transference to the spouse; and how relevant is it to the problems?

Transference is not always a bad thing, and I think to determine that is of interest.

I want to make one last point about a different issue. You made mention of an example by Minuchin, where he dealt with the patient's erotic transference by being antagonistic and hostile to her, and this drove her into her husband's arms. I know you just mentioned this example in passing, and it may be unfair to pick on it, but as it was provocative to me, I am going to do so. There is some question about the ends and the means of this type of therapy.

Sometimes we have to ask ourselves, "Do the ends always justify the means?" "What is the ethical implication of what we are doing in some of the paradoxes?"

I do not mean to bad-mouth paradoxes in total, but I think there are some questions that have to be asked; because in the absence of good outcome data, as we know, all marital therapy suffers. We have to be careful, because we may momentarily, or even a bit longer, drive a spouse into another spouse's arms, but I do not know how long that change lasts. What occurs to me is: What kind of basic human experience has that couple had with the therapist, if paradoxes or that kind are used? I cannot let that go by without voicing my concern.

Dr. Guttman: I think, Michael, you have just emphasized what I have talked about, the difference between transference and transference reaction. I would like to use a different word for what walks into the office—it is not transference; transference should be reserved for the therapist–patient relationship. But, I think, you make another important point, which is between what you call transference reaction, which may arise quickly, and de-transference, which you claim will be worked through in long-term couple therapy. My own sense of that is that couple and family therapy produce very quick results and the results are interactional; they sometimes have feedbck effects on the intrapsychic. If you want to go further, as it were, into intrapsychic characterological phenomena, you change your frame of operation and, of course, in changing your frame of operation you move into classical, real transferential work; but I do not think we should confuse these two dimensions.

Dr. Rosenbluth: My point is not that I agree that in couple therapy the interactional communication work is the basic work. I think, when transference occurs more formally in a longer-term treatment, it should not be the main modality of change; I do not believe it is in individual psychotherapy. In psychoanalysis maybe it is one of the things, but it is a different thing; so, I do not disagree with you and I would not want to imply that. My point is that where transference develops more fully, it sometimes needs to be addressed when it is relevant in terms of impeding the treatment alliance or when it is relevant to what is happening; it is not a substitute for primary focus for the interactional work. So, I really quite agree with you in that way.

Dr. Cameron: I was very surprised when Dr. Guttman said she was not an analyst, because she talks so creatively about countertransference and transference; countertransference in psychoanalysis may not be a surprise, because she talks so clearly about transference. I am interested in the issue of consultation, which, I think, both Lila Russell and Herta referred to.

What do we do when there is a transference/countertransference problem or any other complicated problem?

I think that one thing we do not talk about enough and do not write about enough is that we need to seek consultation with those 30 percent of cases, or when there is an impasse. I do not think it is at all clear whether transference or countertransference needs to be worked out in all cases; probably it most often does. It seems to me that when we have trouble, often that is where the usefulness of asking for a consultation is certainly underestimated. Hunter says that, in 200 consultations they were asked to see, one of the main obstacles to progress was that there were unrecognized transference/countertransference events going on, and I have just one brief example. Before I went into analysis, I was working with a couple that I was having a great deal of fun and a great deal of struggle with. A psychiatrist friend came to town and I started role playing them; as I took on the role of the patient and role played the patient with my psychiatrist friend, I discovered that although I had been treating this couple for 6 months, the man had the same nickname as my father and, literally, for 6 months I had not been aware of that. Then, of course, I began to realize that there was a real countertransference problem going on, and I was involved in some sort of struggle with him. Here I was, thinking I was a relatively sophisticated therapist, but I had not made that connection, and I think we need to find ways around those impasses.

Dr. Guttman: Could I leave you with one thought? Countertransference, as you know, is not a particularly welcome word in family therapy circles, but I was struck by the stalemate. One of the functions of the group is to have an orgy of hatred against the impossible family, or some impossible member, and then you can get down to useful work. The consultative process permits you to have an orgy, an orgy of hatred or whatever it is that you have, and then you get that all out of the way. There are some cases where you cannot do that, because it is too close to home, and two people form a group; you and one person can talk as a group.

Chapter 8

THE RELATIONSHIP OF SEXUAL THERAPY TO MARITAL THERAPY IN PSYCHIATRIC PRACTICE

Edward M. Waring
and
Linden F. Frelick

Psychiatrists who assess and treat couples with relationship problems will find couples who present with specific sexual dysfunction. These couples may reveal sexual dysfunction during the course of marital therapy or may be identified due to failure to progress in therapy because of unresolved sexual problems. Some couples may wish to improve sexual aspects of their marriage as a consequence of successful therapy. This chapter will attempt to describe and address these issues as they relate to marital therapy in psychiatric practice.

This chapter will not be a description of the assessment approach to couples with explicit sexual problems as this is available elsewhere.[1] We will not attempt to describe the functioning of a sexual dysfunction clinic. The chapter will not be a review of basics of sexual counseling and therapy which are well described elsewhere.[2,3,4,5]

The chapter will address the interface between marital conflict and sexual dysfunction in psychiatric practice and develop a typology of marital dysfunction that interacts with overt or covert sexual dysfunction.[6,7] We will describe a method of assessment that when incorporated into the marital assessment in psychiatric practice can detect sexual dysfunction that may initiate, precipitate, or sustain marital discord. We will offer suggestions for treatment of sexual dysfunction detected or revealed during the course of marital therapy.

INTRODUCTION

Masters and Johnson noted that in 44% of couples referred to them, both partners had sexual dysfunction.[15] In the majority of these cases, there was no evidence of primary relationship problems other than the specific symptoms of sexual dysfunction. They point out that sexual dysfunction need not be a symptom of psychiatric disorder, but is often due to poor education, misunderstanding, or a negative attitude.

It seems clear that there is a shift in attitudes among men and women that affects many elements of the marital interaction. The traditional values of sex for procreation and the traditional values of male and female roles all appear to be in transformation. Sexual activity is being perceived more as part of recreation and pleasure. It is clear that the sexual interaction as part of the male/female equilibrium has connections with changing roles, intimacy, power, how affects are handled, and has a relationship to issues of dependency within the relationship. It is clear then that the marital unit may function at a much more complicated level with changing expectations reflecting shifts from the traditional marriage. These shifts may manifest problems, both for the male and female member of the unit.

In a recent study by Anderson and Ruperstein[14] of couples who felt they have effective marriages, 80% reported their marital and sexual relations were happy and satisfying. However, 40% of the men reported erectile or ejaculatory dysfunction and 63% of the women reported arousal or orgasmic dysfunction.

The connection between the marital discord and sexual dysfunction is the factor that influences the course of treatment. If the sexual dysfunction results in marital discord, sex therapy would be the treatment of choice. Sex therapy is not the treatment of choice when sexual dysfunction is the result of marital discord. Marital therapy might be the choice of treatment and often results in improvement in the sexual relationship.

While it is a truism that for many couples the quality of the marital relationship is mirrored in the quality of the sexual relationship, and vice versa, for many other couples a good relationship does not guarantee a satisfactory sexual functioning, and we have seen couples with severe discord whose one area of satisfaction is in the bedroom. Research has shown that sexual dysfunction and marital stress may operate independently of one another.[6] Thus, effective treatment of marital discord may be neither a necessary nor a sufficient condition for improvement in sexual functioning.

Sager has suggested that marital and sex therapy are clinically interrelated in most cases because they deal with different symptoms of overlapping aspects of the couple's total relationship.[8] The connection between the marital discord and the sexual dysfunction is the factor that influences the course of treatment. Sex therapy is not the treatment of choice when severe discord precludes the possibility of good sexual functioning. Anderson and Kupfer found that couples seeking marital therapy had a similar degree of sexual difficulties as a group of couples seeking sex therapy, but the relationships in the marital group were antagonistic compared to the affectionate relationships in the sex therapy group.[9]

Our research on marital intimacy sheds some light on the relationship of the quality of sex to the quality of the relationship.[10] We have consistently found that in the general population, respondents note sexuality as not being a major factor in their level of intimacy.[11] Wives generally report less sexual fulfillment in their marriages than their husbands; husbands see their sexual relationship as a separate component of their marriage relationship, while wives associate their sexual relationship with their level of intimacy. Responding in a socially desirable manner is an important component of assessing intimacy. These findings suggest couples may be reluctant to reveal sexual dysfunction in marital assessment because of different perceptions in social desirability.

We will now describe a method for screening for sexual dysfunction in marital assessment, and then use case illustrations to address issues related to the management of sexual dysfunction as it is presented during marital therapy in psychiatric practice.

MARITAL ASSESSMENT

We have previously described a method of marital assessment that involves gathering information about the couples' complaints, their theories of why the problems developed, a history of their relationship from their first meeting to the present, their observations of their parents' relationships, and their current functioning as a couple.[12]

This allows several opportunities for the couple to reveal information about sexual dysfunction. It is unusual that sexual dysfunction is the presenting complaint, but it may be mentioned as a consequence of the problem. Occasionally, when asked to explain the development of the problem, a spouse may refer to sexual dysfunction. A common example would be a couple whose presenting problem is lack of communication. When asked their theories about this lack of communication, a spouse may disclose that his wife won't speak to him since his affair. When asked what motivated the affair, a sexual dysfunction may be revealed.

A second opportunity to detect sexual dysfunction comes when gathering data about the developmental history of the relationship, including questions about attraction, dating, courtship, and the honeymoon. When asking about the honeymoon, it is easy to ask about the quality of the sexual relationship because this is a period where socially acceptable sexual activity may commence. Of course, many couples will reveal that sexual activity preceded the marriage, but more inhibited couples are given the opportunity to describe sexual dysfunction that may have been present since marriage or even before. Often the couple will be surprised to relate sexual dysfunction that has been accepted for years as status quo in the relationship.

The third opportunity to detect sexual dysfunction comes when you assess the quality of the current relationship, including questions about affection, conflict resolution, commitment, expressiveness, and, of course, sexuality. These opportunities may reveal only that the marital partners are reluctant to disclose information or appear uncomfortable with the questions. In this case, couples are given self-report questionnaires, which include questions about sexual dysfunction, to complete on their own and return later.

If one or more of these opportunities for detection of sexual dysfunction is positive, or if the presenting problem is a sexual attitude or behavior, then, obviously, a complete sexual history is indicated. Several authors have provided summaries of techniques of interviewing and data gathering that constitute a complete sexual history, and these will not be repeated here although we would like to make several comments.[1,2,3,4,5]

Interviewing Couples with Marital Discord—Hints Suggesting Sexual Dysfunction

We will give some examples of responses during marital assessment which should alert the interviewer to the possibility of sexual dysfunction.

A common response to a question about what attracted an individual to his/her future spouse is, "He was a gentleman," or, "He wasn't after just one thing," or, "She was a lady." Although these responses do not have to be followed up, they often do reveal a discomfort with the individual's own sexuality or attitudes at the time of courtship. This may represent a compatibility in low sexual desire in the couple or a specific conflict. For example, a woman may have liked the fact that her husband was not sexually aggressive at first but after 6 months of dating was disturbed that he never made a pass at her and wondered if he was homosexual. When she mentioned this, he became more sexually attentive, but since the wedding sexual activity has diminished. Obviously, a more complete sexual history would be necessary at this time. Another common history would be a man who respected his girlfriend's discomfort with his sexual advances because he assumed that she wanted to retain her virginity until marriage. However, on the honeymoon he discovered that she was not really interested in sex and had had a previous traumatic sexual experience.

Both of these examples show that many couples do not disclose their attitudes, values, preferences, or behaviors regarding sexuality during courtship. The absence of self-disclosure may be a general factor that affects all aspects of a couple's relationship or it may be specifically limited to sexuality. Occasionally, a marital assessment interview may be the first opportunity for a couple to disclose sexual dysfunction.

A second opportunity to assess sexual attitudes, values, and behaviors comes with questions about the honeymoon. A question such as "How was your honeymoon?" allows the interviewer to assess the couple's comfort with discussing their sexuality. Some couples will respond to the above question with a travel itinerary, and some will respond with sexual information. Further probes, such as, "Most people think of honeymoons as a time for sexual adjustment or discovery," allows the couple a general stimulus to disclose information. All interviewers are alert to brief responses, such as, "Sex is OK," or, "Everything was fine," which possibly indicate that everything was not so good. A few specific questions about enjoyment, frequency, or problems may be indicated at this time.

While gathering data about the couple's history, it is important to obtain details about the birth of children. It is worthy to note how frequently the birth of a child is during a time of significant change in both marital quality and sexual functioning. Belsky and Isabella have shown that in the general population there is a significant but moderate decrease in marital satisfaction after the birth of the first child.[13] This also occurs frequently with couples seeking marital therapy, but particularly an increase in sexual dysfunction appears at this time. The most common issue is not only a decrease in the frequency of intercourse but also in the quality of sexual activity.

Finally, when we assess the current relationship, we again focus on sexuality but now with the advantage of some knowledge about the couple's comfort with disclosing information, their attitudes and values, and specific behaviors and satisfactions. With the above desensitization, it is appropriate to ask about specific issues—orgasm, ejaculation, extramarital sex, or even paraphilias. Despite the above screening, about 10% to 20% of couples fail to disclose pertinent information about sexual dysfunction, although in some of these cases there is a suspicion that the couples are not being candid.

Now, we will describe some cases that illustrate the role of sexual dysfunction and therapy in marital therapy in psychiatric practice.

CASE HISTORY #1

The first case is an example of a couple who have sought marital counseling, but sexual dysfunction becomes apparent during the assessment interview.

The couple arrived 15 to 20 minutes late for the appointment. She appeared very tense, and he looked somewhat effeminate. They were a professional couple in their late thirties, with no children. They apologized profusely for being late and stated that they had poor communication and arguments for the past 2 years. He said this was all his fault because he was going through a mid-life crisis. He had seen a psychiatrist for individual counseling during this period. She said she did not know what was troubling him at the time but he seemed depressed.

They met while at professional school and said they had had a friendship for a year because they were both too busy for romance. She described her parents' marriage as poor, and they separated when she was quite young. He said his parents had a stable marriage, but the home atmosphere was oppressively strict and demanding.

After drifting apart for a year, he heard that she had returned from abroad and had some difficulties so he called to help. Their friendship was renewed, and they were very vague about their motives for marriage. When asked about romance, he disclosed that they had had intercourse once and so he felt obliged to marry her. When asked about her sexual functioning, she began to cry and revealed that about one year ago she had discovered that he was homosexual—this was the focus of their crisis. Because of their lateness, they were invited back to continue their assessment.

In the second interview, he revealed that he had had primarily homosexual fantasies since childhood but had never acted on these fantasies and had never disclosed them to his wife. She denied having any sexual fantasy, and since marriage had had a number of obscure medical problems, which she felt limited their sexual activity, she gradually became quite obese. They revealed they had not had intercourse for 2 years and that they had never really enjoyed their sexuality. They were previously in concurrent marital therapy with a psychiatrist but had not chosen to reveal any of this information.

In presenting to them recommendations for therapy, the therapist suggested that the major problem would seem to be a failure to disclose fundamental information to one another during courtship and a contract of living with these secrets during their marriage. It was suggested that these motives be explored before commencing any specific marital or sexual counseling. Their motivations for seeking counseling at this time would have to be carefully assessed. Their reasons for staying together would also have to be clarified.

This case is a good example of how marital discord and sexual dysfunction are often interrelated and overlapping. While there has been sexual dysfunction since the beginning of the marriage, this may be related to a more general lack of disclosure and the absence of honest communication, which may have protected both from dealing with other painful relationship difficulties. It may be impossible to disentangle chicken and egg questions, but it is clear their previous therapy was ineffective because the sexual dysfunction was withheld, and the screening will allow a more comprehensive assessment of what therapy, if any, is indicated for this couple.

CASE HISTORY #2

This couple was a professional couple in their thirties, with two daughters, ages 15 and 10. Their presenting problem was persistent arguments about parenting the girls, particularly the oldest girl. The wife considered the husband fussy, critical, and unsupportive, and he considered her interfering and unwilling to assert discipline.

The history revealed that they had met at work, she had not liked him at first, and one of her coworkers let him know this. This led to conversation, which led him to offer her a ride to and from work. She was attracted to him because he was very shy and not sexually aggressive, and he found her attractive and a good companion. He disclosed that he had been raised in a very strict, undemonstrative family. She said her parents' marriage was stable but that there were issues of family members being unpopular and harassed in their neighborhood. They denied any specific sexual difficulties, but there was a suggestion of some unpleasant sexual experience in her past. They attributed their lack of current sexual interest to bitterness about the arguments and poor communication. They agreed to 10 sessions involving self-disclosure to try to understand their difficulty to resolve conflict.

This couple did extremely well in therapy, and after only three sessions recognized that their power conflict was demonstrating to the daughter how a man and woman who are bitterly disappointed with love might behave in a way that reveals an unspoken message to never fall in love. They were advised to go out on a date together and specifically tell their daughter they were leaving her at home because they wanted romantic time for themselves.

They reported in session four that they had done this and how much better they were getting along. They seemed to recognize that they had a marriage in which the arguments were between that part of himself that was like his fussy mother and that part of herself that was like her interfering mother. They were asked their theories about the quality of the sex life these two women would enjoy if they were married to each other. They thought this was funny and agreed that it would be lousy because they would be inhibited.

In session four they also disclosed that she had been anorgasmic, and he suffered with premature ejaculation since the start of their marriage. She revealed that she had been sexually molested by a relative, and he had been a virgin when they married. They had no language to communicate their sexual needs or preferences and were too ashamed to seek counseling.

As part of their marital counseling, they were given information about premature ejaculation and techniques that they might attempt on their own to improve their sexual functioning during the next five sessions; if there was no improvement they would be referred for specific sexual counseling. During the next five weeks, she became orgasmic, and referral was thought by the couple to be unnecessary.

This couple were highly motivated, committed to their marriage, and had a genuine affection for one another. In the course of marital counseling, for lack of communication and inability to resolve differences of opinion, a specific sexual dysfunction was revealed. One could postulate the sexual dysfunction had contributed to the relationship difficulty. The rapid movement in their intimacy, due to increased self-disclosure, led them spontaneously to address their sexual dysfunction with only general information, reading, and knowledge of the squeeze technique for premature ejaculation. The improvement in their relationship allowed the opportunity to successfully address a sexual dysfunction with minimal intervention.

CASE HISTORY #3

This couple, in their late forties, were part of a research project, which they entered because of their 21-year-old son who was diagnosed as schizophrenic. The research program gave the parents the opportunity to learn about the disorder, attend a support group with other parents of schizophrenic children, and have specific marital therapy if they wished.

This couple agreed to participate in 10 sessions to understand how they had drifted apart since she had had a mastectomy and to effectively handle their difficulties in resolving differences of opinion about their son.

During the course of the therapy, it was disclosed that the husband had experienced symptoms of obsessive-compulsive neurosis during their courtship. He had grave doubts about getting married. When the wife found herself pregnant he felt resentful that the good times were over, and she resented that she had to give up a promising career. The boy had had a series of difficulties, including being a colicky baby; he had school phobia and was subsequently truant and he engaged in minor antisocial behavior. These difficulties split the parents: she saw the problem as caused by his lack of disciplining his son, and he thought she was overindulgent.

Two years ago she had had a mastectomy, and after the operation they had been unable to talk about the consequences. He disclosed that shortly before the operation he had his first episode of impotence.

After completion of their marital therapy which had led to a decrease in their arguments, increased communication, and increased feelings of closeness, they were referred to a sexual dysfunction clinic. A 6-month follow-up revealed they were sexually active again without sexual dysfunction.

This couple became involved in marital therapy in response only to their desire to give their son, who was being treated for a psychiatric disorder, proper and adequate aftercare. The marital therapy was focused on issues of difficulty in their relationship related to their commitment to the marriage from its inception, and current problems with conflict resolution and lack of affection. In the course of therapy, a specific sexual dysfunction was disclosed which did not improve spontaneously with modest improvements in their marital relationship. Referral to and treatment in a sexual dysfunction clinic resulted in the successful treatment of an impotence problem, with generalized improvement in their marriage. Their son is doing well with outpatient follow-up on a minimum dose of a major tranquilizer.

CASE HISTORY #4

This couple, in their twenties and married for one year, were referred to a research project on the treatment of depressed married women. She had been seen for three sessions by a psychiatrist, with a diagnosis of a major affective disorder, and had been receiving an adequate dose of an antidepressant medication without response.

The couple stated that they were very much in love and had a good relationship except for sexual difficulties present since the honeymoon. She had been injured in a car accident on the honeymoon, with soft tissue injuries to her neck and back.

They both described their parents' marriages as stable and loving. She suggested that her mother tended to be somewhat domineering. The couple had dated for several years and said they were quite compatible, were good listeners, and were committed to the marriage.

They were both virgins when they married, and this was very important to both in the context of their families and culture. Neither had had any sexual information from their families, and neither had had experience with masturbation. They both enjoyed foreplay, experienced sexual arousal, but she had been anorgasmic since marriage and was still experiencing discomfort from her injuries. They both readily agreed to a referral to a sexual dysfunction clinic.

This couple, although referred for a marital assessment, never attributed her depression or their sexual dysfunction to their relationship. The etiology of the sexual dysfunction will be investigated with possible contributing causes, including sexual knowledge and attitudes, depression, or physical injury.

CASE HISTORY #5

This couple, in their late fifties, were seen for an assessment as a consequence of the husband's failure to respond to treatment for a major affective disorder. He attributed his depression to a failure to perform in his job, the return home of his daughter and grandchildren after a separation, and a poor relationship with his wife. She was originally seen independently and thought to suffer from a major affective disorder with successful response to antidepressants.

The marital assessment began with her discussing that she thought he had had an affair 2 years previously. He denied this, and said that he had simply withdrawn due to her critical attitude.

When asked when the difficulties began, she said 2 years ago, and he said longer than that but could not say when. She attributed the problem to leaving work and being bored. He attributed the problem to feeling isolated and a lack of affection.

In their first session, he attributed the onset of their difficulties to the birth of their first child. He believed she became preoccupied with her role as mother. She attributed their difficulties to his less attentive manner towards her right after the wedding, being preoccupied with his career.

In their second session, they disclosed that she had been anorgasmic since the honeymoon and that he had premature ejaculation. They had both gradually withdrawn with considerable bitterness.

In their third session, she disclosed that all the girls in her family had been quite lustful and had had many boyfriends, husbands, and sexual experiences. He disclosed that his family was preoccupied with sexual humor, and raised the possibility of incest.

This couple provides an example of a common pattern of early sexual dysfunction becoming a focus of chronic marital discord. Therapy focused initially on resolving this mutual bitterness which prevented any specific behavioral attempts to improve sexual functioning. One assumes the sexual dysfunction played some role in his failure to respond to other treatment approaches.

DISCUSSION

If these cases are representative of the types of sexual dysfunction that marital therapists will encounter, what are the implications for the relationship of sexual therapy to marital discord in cases that are referred to psychiatrists?

First, psychiatrists and other mental health professionals should recognize that simple or unifocal approaches to all couples will be unsuccessful for a significant number of clients, not because of client response but because of the professionals' failure to appreciate the necessity for applying principles of differential therapeutics and meeting patient expectations. Successful treatment of couples with marital discord and sexual dysfunction will always involve combinations of education, counseling, psychotherapy, behavioral approaches, medications, and physical treatments at various times and in various proportions. The psychiatrist must have an appreciation and respect for complexity, a tolerance of ambiguity, and an ability to work with other professionals.

Second, most psychiatrists will not be trained in marital therapy, sexual counseling, gynecology, or urology which are the basic skills. We have advocated that the basic skills for the marital therapist are detection, preliminary assessment, and referral practices. Of course, some may also wish to gain training and experience in sexual counseling.

REFERENCES

1. Watters, W.W., Akswith, J., Cohn, M., & Lamont, J.A. (1985). An assessment approach to couples with sexual problems. *Canadian Journal of Psychiatry, 30,* 2–11.
2. Kaplan, H.S. (1983). *The evaluation of sexual disorders: Psychological and medical aspects.* New York: Brunner/Mazel.
3. Lo Piccolo, J., & Lo Piccolo, L. (1978). *Handbook of sex therapy.* New York: Plenum Press.
4. Hawton, K. (1985). *Sex therapy: A practical guide.* Toronto: Oxford University Press.
5. Green, R. (1980). *Human sexuality: A health practitioners text.* (2nd ed.). Baltimore: Williams & Wilkins.
6. Hartman, L.M. (1980). The interface between sexual dysfunction and mental conflict. *American Journal of Psychiatry, 137* (5):576–579.
7. Roffe, M.W., & Britt, B.C. (1981). A typology of marital interaction for sexually dysfunctional couples. *Journal of Sexual and Marital Therapy, 7,* 207–222.
8. Sager, C.J. (1976). The role of sex therapy in marital therapy. *American Journal of Psychiatry, 133,* 555–559.
9. Anderson, F.E., & Kupfer, D.J. (1976). Profiles of couples seeking sex therapy and marital therapy. *American Journal of Psychiatry, 133,* 559–562.
10. Patton, D., Waring, E.M. (1985). Sex and marital intimacy. *Journal of Sexual and Marital Therapy, 11*(3):176–184.

11. Waring, E.M., Tillman, M.P., Frelick, L., Russell, L., & Weisz, G. (1980). Concepts of intimacy in the general population. *Journal of Nervous and Mental Disorders, 168*(8):471–474.
12. Waring, E.M. (1981). Facilitating marital intimacy through self disclosure. *American Journal of Family Therapy, 9*(4):33–42.
13. Belsky, J., & Isabella, R.A. (1985). Marital and parent-child relationships in family of origin and marital change following the birth of a baby: A retrospective analysis. *Child Development, 56*(2):342–349.
14. Anderson, F.E., & Ruperstein, C. (1978). Frequency of sexual dysfunction in normal couples. *New England Journal of Medicine, 299,* 111–115.
15. Masters, W., & Johnson, V. (1966). *Human sexual response.* Boston: Little, Brown.

Chapter 9

COMBINED THERAPIES

Edward M. Waring

The term "combined therapy" was introduced by Greene and Solomon in 1963[1] to refer to the mixing of conjoint and concurrent sessions. *Concurrent marital therapy* is the modality in which the therapist sees each spouse separately, and *conjoint marital therapy* is the practice of seeing both spouses together during all therapeutic sessions. The authors advocated this approach as providing information that might not be disclosed with the spouse present. This approach allowed the therapist in the conjoint session to assess whether the impressions disclosed were distortions or accurate perceptions. These authors suggested that combining these two approaches increased rapport between the couple and therapist. Critics of the combined approach suggested that disclosures in the individual sessions often constituted secrets that made conjoint sessions impossible. The critics suggested that combining these approaches produced confusion, not clarification. This debate, based on different therapists' varying clinical experience, remains unresolved and is perhaps unresolvable. Few authors today write about their experiences with combined therapy although it is often practiced.

In this paper, the definition of combined therapy will be broadened from the concept introduced by Greene and Solomon to include the combination of marital therapy with any other specific therapeutic modality, including individual therapy, behavior therapy, group therapy, sexual therapy, family therapy, and drug therapy. I will review works that have attempted to systematically evaluate combined therapies as opposed to those in which authors advocate their approach as superior to others, based solely on their clinical experience.

As a focus, it will be assumed that all therapy is combined therapy although the elements that are combined are not always explicit. For example, in one case where the mother had made her second serious suicide attempt, the family was assessed. The interview focused on an older son who was frustrated that he had to run the family business and who was concerned about his younger brother who was abusing drugs and involved in much mischief. As the interview proceeded, the parents were noted to be sitting together on the couch, both hunched over in a typical depressive posture. After questioning that revealed major affective disorders in both spouses, it was suggested that both parents might benefit from a trial of antidepressant medication, monitored by the oldest son. Two weeks later they were a different family. The father had assumed responsibility for the business, the couple were spontaneous and bright, the younger son had stopped acting out, and the older boy was relieved. One wonders whether it was the family assessment, the medication, the combination, or some other unknown factor that produced this dramatic result.

Another couple who were referred because of a possible divorce as a result of the husband's affair, showed the wife assuming a position of moral superiority and castigating her husband with self-justified outrage which he readily accepted and even encouraged. She was a born-again Christian and he expressed that he deserved to suffer for his sins. During the next two sessions, the therapist attempted to help them understand factors in their relationship that might have contributed to the affair, but they appeared to want to continue the pattern of his punishment under her verbal attacks. The therapist did not recognize the couple who arrived for the fourth session. The husband had become a born-again Christian and the couple was obviously content. What combination of therapy would have been so rapidly effective in this case?

While we prefer to believe clinical improvement is a consequence of either our specific therapy or characteristics of ourselves as therapists, a variety of other factors, both specific and nonspecific, influence outcome.

Let us review *opinions* expressed about the combination of marital therapy with other therapeutic modalities. Reviewed will be the outcome studies that have specifically evaluated marital therapy with other therapies in specific disorders. Also discussed will be the theoretical and clinical implications of combined therapies.

In addition, the writer will describe his clinical experience with combined therapies and will use his clinical experience to comment on the literature that he has reviewed. Where appropriate, observations that consistently appear in the literature will be emphasized.

Third, the writer will present a summary of a recent research project on the effectiveness of combining marital therapy with antidepressant medication in the treatment of major affective disorder in married women. Finally, the writer will suggest several possibilities for clinical outcome research on combined therapies and present a summary of existing knowledge on combined marital therapy.

THE COMBINATION OF MARITAL THERAPY AND INDIVIDUAL THERAPY

Since psychoanalysis was the predominant approach to therapy in the 1940s and since psychoanalysis focused on conflicts within individuals, it is not surprising that in the early psychiatric writings *concurrent marital therapy*, in which the therapist saw each spouse separately, was described first by Mittleman.[2] Many other nonpsychiatric professionals were already involved in what was largely referred to as *marital counseling*, involving conjoint sessions with both spouses. The psychiatrist's early rationale was that the *transference* relationship between patient and therapist was essential to the therapeutic cure. The presence of a spouse during the therapeutic hour would inevitably present reality conflicts that would disrupt this relationship. By analyzing both partners, the therapist was thought to be in a better position to observe which marital interaction problems were reality determined and which were neurotically determined.[2]

The most significant trend in marital therapy since that time has been the increased importance placed on working with the marital relationship per se and not only with the individuals in the relationship. Cookerly[4] suggests this choice is largely determined by the theoretical bias of the therapist. Those therapists who view distress as due to personal maladjustment would recommend individual or concurrent sessions. Therapists who believe distress is due to insufficient social skills would suggest conjoint group sessions. Those who view marital maladjustment as an entity in and of itself would advocate conjoint sessions. Unfortunately, this analogy suggests that only those therapists without opinions or who are confused about their theoretical bias would suggest combined therapy as defined by Greene and Solomon. Nowhere in the literature does it suggest that client expectations or therapist experience or skills might influence the choice of therapy. No authors report that combined therapy is ineffective in their experience.

The practice of seeing both spouses together during all therapeutic sessions has come to be known as *conjoint marital therapy*. The mixing of conjoint and concurrent sessions became known as *combined marital therapy*. The use of two therapists, each seeing a spouse separately and then consulting together, became commonly known as *collaborative therapy*. *Collaborative combined therapy* involves the use of separate therapists for each spouse with all four people meeting together at regular intervals for joint sessions.

All possible combinations and permutations of concurrent, conjoint, collaborative, and combined consecutive techniques have been practiced. What have we learned about the effectiveness of each of these methods? Surprisingly little! There have been *no* adequate experiments that have tested whether working with both spouses, either concurrently or conjointly, is more efficient, effective, or humane, than working with only one troubled spouse in individual therapy. Gurman and Kniskern[3] in their review of marital therapy outcome research, suggest that there is tentative evidence that conjoint marital therapy appears to be as effective or possibly more effective than individual therapy for a wide variety of interpersonal marital problems. However, there is no evidence to support the superiority of conjoint over combined therapy. Gurman and Kniskern's conclusion is based on 44 comparative studies, 31 of which reported that conjoint marital therapy methods were reported as superior in comparison to individual therapy, communication training, or verbal counseling. Gurman and Kniskern claim that the limited evidence on the application of individual therapy to marital problems produces a deterioration rate of about 12%. However, no studies of combined therapy have been reported.

These rather gross estimates should be considered in relation to a number of facts. First, most of the research is uncontrolled. Second, the type of marital therapy is rarely explicit. Third, the types of problems for which the couple has usually sought help are usually not the kinds of difficulties that come to the attention of psychiatrists. And fourth, the marital therapy sessions are usually very brief and the methodological designs are usually extremely limited.

In light of the above, the best data on the subject are from the pilot study by Cookerly in 1973.[4] He surveyed the follow-up records of 773 former marital clients of 21 marriage counselors. He divided the outcomes into six groups: clients who remained married with poor, moderate, or good outcome and clients who divorced with poor, moderate, or good outcome. He also divided the forms of therapy into six basic practices:

1. Individual therapy with only one spouse.
2. Individual group therapy with only one spouse.
3. Concurrent individual therapy.
4. Concurrent groups.
5. Conjoint therapy.
6. Conjoint groups.

Obviously, combined therapy was not evaluated!

The most striking results were as follow. Conjoint therapy was most successful for those couples who remained married, but produced the poorest outcome for those who obtained divorces. Conjoint groups ranked second for couples remaining married and first for those obtaining divorces. Individual interviews were worse for those remaining married, but second best for those obtaining divorces. *Concurrent therapy*, which was the most common marital therapy at the time, was *worst* overall, ranking last for those who remained married and second to last for those who obtained divorces. Should the worst type of marital therapy be combined with anything?

The problem with these data is that the results are as

inadequate as they are provocative. The study was not a controlled experiment but rather a pilot survey, and no definitive study followed. As a result, the many uncontrolled variables confound the data and make meaningful conclusions impossible. Cookerly went on to compare these therapies on measures of client attitudes, client follow-up, and psychometric tests. He concluded that best results were obtained for conjoint interview, but if divorce, unhappy outcomes or social skills training were expected, then *conjoint group* was the best alternative. Concurrent therapy uniformly led to the worst outcome.

Beck[5] reports on the Family Service Associate of America census by interview and/or questionnaire of 1,257 clients where the marriage was the primary problem. She concluded that patients treated by conjoint interviews showed significantly higher change scores than did those treated mainly with individual interviews.

In summary, conjoint therapy is now practiced almost exclusively, and concurrent and collaborative approaches are rarely mentioned. Combined therapy has been advocated, but was never evaluated, and today is seldom discussed.

COMBINED MARITAL THERAPY AND GROUP THERAPY

As group therapy grew in popularity and respectability so too did the use of groups for married couples. Treating spouses in separate groups became known as *concurrent group therapy* while when spouses together participated in the same group this was termed *conjoint group therapy*. The method of bringing couples together in groups led by other couples was created by Ely[6] and called *conjugal therapy*. Marital groups have also varied in composition, being made up of all couples with one therapist, of all couples with cotherapists, and of couples placed together with unmarried patients.

Cookerly's research again showed that conjoint groups rank second for couples who remain married and first for those obtaining divorces. Again, what is striking is the absence of any kind of outcome that can tell us anything about the effectiveness, efficiency, or humaneness of these therapies.

THE COMBINATION OF MARITAL THERAPY AND BEHAVIOR THERAPY

Jacobson's[7] review of the research on the effectiveness of marital therapy suggests strongly that those therapies based on theories of behavioral change and communication have the strongest support in controlled outcome trials in terms of therapeutic efficacy. However, the combination of a specific marital therapy and a specific form of behavior therapy has not been reported up to this time.

However, there have been a number of well-controlled trials of spouse-aided behavior therapy in the treatment of obesity and agoraphobia that suggest that this is an effective treatment modality. Weisz and Bucher[8] and later Brownell and co-workers[9] have demonstrated that using the spouse to actively reinforce weight reduction behavior in females produces better weight reduction and weight maintenance, improved marital functioning, and decrease of depression in the overweight spouse in comparison to control groups where the spouse is passively involved. This is similar to the work of Hafner[10] with patients with agoraphobia where the spouse is again actively involved in the reinforcement paradigm, with improved results over control situations. Although this is not a specific combination of a specific marital therapy technique with a specific behavioral technique, it would appear that spouse-aided behavioral techniques are clearly efficacious in certain specific disorders such as obesity and agoraphobia. Cobb and co-workers[11] have recently published a report that questions the efficacy of combining marital therapy with behavior therapy in agoraphobia.

MARITAL THERAPY AND FAMILY THERAPY

Gurman[12] analyzed 118 mostly uncontrolled studies of marital and family therapy in which an estimate was made of improvement rates. Overall, the different types of nonbehavioral marital therapies produced improvement rates of 61 to 65 percent, which is comparable to those produced by nonmarital individual therapy.

However, again it is striking that no one has ever done an outcome study of the combination of marital therapy and family therapy. Individual clinical reports suggest that therapists switch from one modality to the other in separate sessions or within the context of the family sessions with great regularity, depending on their orientation. There have, however, been no studies that actively compare family therapy alone with marital therapy alone or a combination of marital and family therapy for similar problems.

Our own research on *cognitive family therapy* may have some relevance in addressing this theoretical issue. In cognitive family therapy, an initial family assessment with all family members is done, but subsequently only the married couple is seen for 10 one-hour sessions over a 10-week period. In five different types of outcome research we have demonstrated that cognitive family therapy is an effective form of therapy in reducing symptoms of nonpsychotic emotional illness in one or both spouses, increasing marital adjustment, and improving measures of family function and environment. However, no comparison has actually been made with the same group of families when all family members were present in all sessions. The opportunity to evaluate such an outcome in a disorder such as anorexia nervosa, with hospitalized patients being assigned randomly, one group to family therapy and one group to cognitive family therapy, would be an ideal paradigm for evaluating the combination, and for suggesting answers to questions such as when and in what situations one should switch from one type of therapy to another.

COMBINED MARITAL THERAPY AND DRUG THERAPY

There are two outcome studies, one by Friedman[13] in the treatment of outpatient neurotic depression that combined marital therapy and antidepressant medication, and one by Leff and co-workers[14] in which phenothiazines were combined with a form of marital therapy designed to reduce expressed emotion. These two studies showed that combined marital therapy and drug therapy are additive in effect. Leff and co-workers' study, however, combined family therapy and marital therapy and it is difficult to sort out the difference between the two.

Davenport[15] in a series of studies compared the outcome of 14 patients with manic-depressive illness who participated in conjoint marital group therapy with 53 patients who refused. All patients were receiving follow-up care with lithium. The group that had no marital therapy had significantly more relapses, hospitalizations, and divorces. Selection factors obviously obscured these results. Davenport suggests such groups have important implications for social support, early detection, education, and treatment adherence.

In summary, there is only one study in the entire literature, that by Freidman,[13] that uses an adequate research design to evaluate the combination of marital therapy with another therapeutic modality. In this one study on neurotically depressed outpatients, the combination was additive, but it is clear that the antidepressant medication had its major effect on depressive symptomatology, and that the marital therapy had its major effect on the quality of the interpersonal marital relationships.

In summary, there are many problems that remain in doing outcome studies in combined therapy, which include:

1. Difficulty in providing long-term control groups.
2. Inappropriate exposure of often unmotivated patients to psychiatric treatment.
3. High dropout rates.
4. Highly heterogeneous patients.
5. Lack of standardization of the marital therapy being offered.
6. Inadequate outcome measures.

As well as these technical difficulties, which are less of an obstacle now than they were a decade ago, the following philosophical questions need to be addressed: What are the overall therapeutic benefits of marital therapy alone on the patients with a specific disorder? What are the overall therapeutic benefits of any other type of therapy on the same group of patients with the same disorders? What kinds of patients are benefited the most from marital therapy alone or the therapy to be combined with marital therapy alone? What kinds of patients benefit most from the combined approach? On what kinds of outcomes does the marital therapy have its greatest effects? What are the general and specific effects of marital therapy in combination with another therapeutic modality? Finally, in regard to the combined effect: (1) is it additive? (2) does it result in potentiation? (3) is it inhibitive? or (4) is it reciprocal?

Karasu[16] suggests in regard to combined therapies that: (1) each may have differential effects or loci of outcome, (2) each is activated and sustained on a different time schedule, and (3) each may best relate to different disorders.

PERSONAL OBSERVATIONS COMBINING MARITAL THERAPY WITH OTHER TREATMENT MODALITIES

Since I have worked in the general hospital setting for the past 10 years, the vast majority of couples I have treated with marital therapy have received marital therapy in combination with some other form of therapeutic intervention. Since patients are often assessed in the inpatient psychiatric unit, in consultations on other floors, in the emergency department, in the outpatient department, and in private outpatient referrals, the majority of patients that I have seen have been referred for problems of an individual psychiatric nature. The patients have usually not had the expectation of a marital assessment or therapy as one of their priorities.

A small proportion of my practice is outpatient private referrals of couples for specific marital assessment and therapy. These marital problems included lack of intimacy, frequent arguments, affairs, and other interpersonal difficulties. I see practically all these patients for conjoint assessment and for conjoint marital therapy. Many outpatients are also referred individually for symptoms of anxiety or depression, but spend most of their time talking about problems related to their marital situation. The majority of these readily accept a marital assessment interview which may or may not go on to conjoint marital therapy.

I have not done concurrent, collaborative, or combined marital therapy. I have found that after a course of conjoint marital therapy, it is relatively easy to shift some patients into individual therapy. On the other hand, I have found it almost impossible after a prolonged period of individual therapy to switch to marital therapy. My experience has been that when a couple is in conjoint therapy and one individual requests individual attention, it is usually to reveal some secret that the individual is not prepared to deal with or to undermine the conjoint therapeutic approach.

The rest of my practice involves patients with diagnoses of schizophrenia, affective disorder, personality disorder, psychosomatic conditions, crises and suicide attempts, and medical problems and these patients are receiving a variety of psychiatric therapies, medical therapies, and individual therapies at the time that marital assessment is done.

The marital assessment in combination with other treatments for these disorders has three obvious benefits in the total management of these patients, which are: (1) education of the spouse regarding the condition of the patient and therapeutic plan, (2) treatment compliance to the other therapeutic regimes being offered, and (3) identification of factors in the marital relationship that may be perpetuating factors in the individual patient's disorders.

The majority of these patients who receive a marital assessment do not go on to conjoint marital therapy sessions because they express no interest in such sessions or because the assessors do not feel that it is indicated in that it might do more harm than good. In general, my clinical observation of the conditions in which the addition of conjoint marital therapy to the other treatment modalities appears to be ineffective, include major affective disorders, which I will be discussing shortly, and chronic alcoholism, although Jacobson[7] suggests more positive results with alcoholism. The conditions in which the couple express an interest in marital conjoint interviews combined with other treatment modalities where this approach seems clinically effective, are psychosomatic disorders, nonpsychotic emotional illness, and some cases of personality disorders, crises, and suicide attempts.

The therapeutic modalities that in my clinical experience are additive, are the combination of marital therapy with: (1) antidepressants for minor depression, (2) phenothiazines in the treatment of schizophrenia, and (3) behavior therapies in sexual, nonpsychotic emotional illness and psychosomatic conditions. The psychosomatic conditions in which the addition of marital therapy to other treatment modalities appears to be most effective, are in the treatment of obesity, hypochondriasis, masked depression, and chronic pain problems.

In summary, my clinical experience to this point suggests that the most fertile area for outcome research involves combining marital therapy with drug and behavioral therapies in the treatment of nonpsychotic emotional illnesses, psychosomatic and medical conditions, and sexual dysfunctions.

I will now attempt to combine the literature with my clinical experience to suggest some general guidelines regarding combined marital therapies:

1. While there is no evidence regarding the effectiveness, efficiency, or humaneness of combining individual and marital therapy, clinical experience has resulted in the majority of therapists using the conjoint approach with problems of marital adjustment. Since the most effective therapies are structured and focus on direct communication, it is relatively efficient and humane to initiate therapy from a conjoint model and shift to individual and/or group if the conjoint sessions are proving ineffective, divorce appears imminent, or severe psychopathology interferes.

2. The combination of spouse-assisted behavioral therapies for sexual dysfunctions, psychosomatic conditions, and nonpsychotic emotional illness is well established, and clinical experience and research will establish which types of combined therapies are most effective in specific disorders.

3. The issue of combining marital therapy with family therapy remains of considerable theoretical and clinical importance. It is possible that minor changes in marital quality may produce major changes in family function and environment.

4. The combination of drugs and marital therapy is de-

veloping specific clinical indications and contraindications. In dysthymic depressions, the combination of antidepressants and marital therapy is additive; in major affective disorders in women, antidepressants alone are better in the acute phase; and in manic-depressive disorders it would appear that the combination of lithium and conjoint group marital therapy improves the prognosis. Research on the major and minor tranquilizers is indicated.

SUMMARY

The efficacy of combined therapy, as defined by Greene and Solomon,[1] has never been studied. One assumes clinical experience has led to the predominance of the conjoint approach. Conjoint marital group therapy has also grown in popularity but outcome research is lacking.

The combination of marital therapy with behavior therapy in the treatment of psychosomatic conditions, sexual dysfunctions, and agoraphobia appears to be a promising development.

Friedman's study[13] demonstrated that marital therapy and antidepressants were additive in the treatment of neurotic depression. Our study suggests marital therapy did not improve the outcome for women with major affective disorder treated with antidepressants. Davenport's observations[15] suggest that further evaluation of the combination of lithium and conjoint marital groups in manic-depressives is indicated.

Research is indicated that evaluates outcome in a specific group of patients who receive a specific type of marital therapy in combination with other specific therapies.

COMMENTS ON AN OUTCOME STUDY OF COMBINED THERAPY

I recently completed a study evaluating the combination of antidepressant drugs and marital therapy on the treatment of married women with major affective disorder as defined by Research Diagnostic Criteria.[17] We attempted to replicate Friedman's study which demonstrated the combination of antidepressants and marital therapy was additive in the treatment of outpatients with dysthymic depression.[13] We had completed a short study that demonstrated that deficiencies of marital intimacy were strongly correlated with severity of symptoms of major depression in women.[13] We hypothesized that cognitive family therapy, which is designed to enhance marital intimacy, might be appropriate to combine with antidepressants. Several comments about this study may illuminate the issues discussed previously about combined therapy.

Originally 57 women with a diagnosis of major affective disorder were eligible to participate in the study. Thirty women and their spouses refused to give an informed consent to participate in the research. The most common reason was the unwillingness or unavailability of the spouse. Many women preferred a specific therapy with a specific therapist. One of the limitations in combined therapy is the expectations of the patient or the couple that a specific approach will be used. The patient or couple's theory of what causes the depression may make a combined treatment unacceptable to one or both spouses. One can only speculate regarding the acceptability of combined therapies to professionals.

Of the 27 couples who started the study, only 13 completed the 10-week trial and 6-month follow-up. Thus of the original 57 patients, only about 20% actually completed the trial. One has to wonder if there are fundamental differences between the couples who participated and those who refused for a variety of reasons. Combined therapy, at least in a research setting, is unacceptable to the majority of couples. The results of the research can hardly be generalized to the total clinical population.

The dropout rate, the rate of separation and divorce, and the outcome as measured by improvement in depressive symptoms was significantly worse in the group who received the combination of antidepressants and cognitive family therapy. The study suggests that a specific marital therapy is not indicated in the treatment of major depressive episodes. Several other recent studies support the general conclusion that marital therapy adds nothing to the effectiveness of antidepressants in the major affective disorders.

What can this study tell us about the issue of combined therapy in general? First, the study suggests that such research is feasible. Second, the study suggests that a specific combination of therapies in a specific disorder was less effective, efficient, and humane than the control condition which was antidepressants plus supportive care. This result was in the opposite direction from the research hypothesis and also the opposite result to what would be expected by therapist bias. I would have hoped a therapy that I helped to develop was effective but the objective results seem to suggest otherwise. However, the study design suggests that a methodology exists that provides objective and valid outcome independent of therapist or observer bias. The study design, which largely employed objective self-report questionnaires could be adapted to any clinical practice of marital therapy.

The benefits of such research to my own clinical practice are immediate. In couples referred for marital therapy, I will screen each spouse for the presence of major affective disorders before commencing therapy. If one or both spouses have a major affective disorder, I will advise them not to make decisions about separation, divorce, or marital therapy until they have had an adequate trial with antidepressant medications. This advice has reduced the number of couples who separate and divorce and also reduced by half the couples who want marital therapy after clinical improvement of depression. Finally, if a couple has failed to improve after 8 to 10 sessions of cognitive family therapy, I again screen the spouses for the presence of major affective disorder which occasionally develops during the course of psychotherapy.

In summary, research on combined therapy in depressed individuals has produced some specific clinical recommendations. (1) The combination of antidepressants and marital therapy is additive in the dysthymic depressions. The drugs seem to relieve symptoms, which seems to allow the marital therapy to improve the relationship. (2) The combination of antidepressants and marital therapy is not additive in major depressions in the acute phase. This suggests either that marital discord is secondary to the depression or that self-disclosure makes depressed patients worse. (3) The combination of lithium and marital group psychotherapy improves the prognosis in at least some manic-depressive patients, probably through increasing the compliance with medication.

REFERENCES

1. Greene, B. L., & Solomon, A. P. (1963). Marital disharmony: Concurrent psychoanalytic therapy of husband and wife by the same psychiatrist. *American Journal of Psychotherapy, 17,* 443–456.
2. Mittelman, B. (1968). The concurrent analysis of married couples. *Psychoanalytic Quarterly, 17,* 182–197.
3. Gurman, A. S., & Kniskern, D. P. (1975). Research on marital and family therapy: Progress, perspective, prospect. In S. L. Garfield & A. E. Bergin (Eds.), *Handbook of psychotherapy and behavior change: An empirical analysis,* (2nd ed.). New York: John Wiley & Sons.
4. Cookerly, J. R. (1973). The outcome of the six major forms of marriage counselling compared: A pilot study. *Journal of Marriage and the Family, 35,* 608–611.
5. Beck, D. F. (1970). *The treatment of marital problems.* New York: Family Service Association of America.
6. Ely, A. L. (1970). *Efficacy of training in conjugal therapy.* Unpublished doctoral thesis, Rutgers University.
7. Jacobson, N. S., Follette, W. C., & Elwood, R. W. (in press). Outcome research in behavioral marital therapy: A methodological and conceptual reappraisal. In K. Halweg & N. S. Jacobson (Eds.), *Marital interaction: Analysis and modification.* New York: Guilford.
8. Weisz, G. M., & Bucher, B. (1980). Involving husbands in treatment

of obesity—effects on weight loss, depression, and marital satisfaction. *Behaviour Therapy, 11,* 643–650.
9. Brownell, K. D., Heckerman, C. L., Westlake, R. J., Hayes, S. C., & Monti, P. M. (1978). The effect of couples training and partner cooperativeness in the behavioral treatment of obesity. *Behavior Research and Therapy, 16,* 323–333.
10. Hafner, R. J. (1977). The husbands of agoraphobic women and their influence on treatment outcome. *British Journal of Psychiatry, 131,* 289–294.
11. Cobb, J. P., Mathews, A. M., Childs-Clarke, A., & Blowers, C. M. The spouse as co-therapist in the treatment of agoraphobia. *British Journal of Psychiatry, 144,* 282–287.
12. Gurman, A. S. (1985). The effects and effectiveness of marital therapy. In A. S. Gurman and D. C. Rice (Eds.), *Couples in conflict.* New York: Jason Aronson.
13. Friedman, A. S. (1975). Interaction of drug therapy with marital therapy in depressive patients. *Archives of General Psychiatry, 32,* 619–637.
14. Leff, J., Kuipers, L., Berkowitz, R., Eberlein-Vries, R., & Sturgeon, D. (1982). A controlled trial of social intervention in the families of schizophrenic patients. *British Journal of Psychiatry, 141,* 121–134.
15. Davenport, Y. B. (1981). Treatment of the married bipolar patient in conjoint couples psychotherapy groups. In M. R. Lonsky (Ed.), *Family therapy and major psychopathology.* New York: Grune & Stratton.
16. Karasu, T. B. (1982). Psychotherapy and pharmacotherapy: Toward an integrative model. *American Journal of Psychiatry, 139*(9), 1102–1113.
17. Spitzer, R. L., Endicott, J. E., & Robins, E. (1978). *Research diagnostic criteria (RDC) for a selected group of functional disorders* (3rd ed.). National Institute of Mental Health Clinical Research Branch Collaborative Program on the Psychobiology of Depression. New York: New York State Psychiatric Institute

DISCUSSION

Ernest W. McCrank, M.D.
(University of Western Ontario)

My first contact with marital therapy was when I was in my first 2 months of residency and I had arranged to see a couple. My staffman found out and gave me a real blast on the telephone and said that I had no business interviewing this couple. Not a good beginning. Today 5 to 10% of the people I see in my practice are couples. I don't want to be flippant in evaluating marital therapy itself, let alone the combination of marital therapy with another therapy, but I wonder if in marital therapy there can ever be such a thing as a true control group. I also wonder if we can really match groups. We can look at things like age, years of marriage, sex, and so on but how do you match for things like the perception, on the part of a couple or an individual person in the marriage, of the seriousness of their own disharmony and what it means to them? It seems to me that in a couple or a family, any enhancement of communication skills is valuable and additive. However, Dr. Waring has pointed out that when treating major affective disorders, this may, in fact, have a negative effect. And then I wonder how timing gets to be an issue here and just as I would think when I was treating diabetic ketoacidosis, I wouldn't think of starting a major diabetic education session with a patient lying there in a semicoma. Maybe that's the issue with acute psychiatric disturbances such as depression. You have to treat those things first. I've also noticed with anorexics that when they're down at such a low weight it's pointless to try to talk to them about why they're so thin or about their relationship to the family until their body weight goes up. Dr. Waring made the point that he thought it was difficult to switch from individual therapy to family therapy or marital therapy if he had been seeing the person for a very long time. In my opinion it's almost impossible.

I see an improvement in the communication of the family as being important, not only to psychiatric disorders but in applying it to medical conditions as well. When I was doing a year of internal medicine, I saw a lady who came in with bilateral tingling in her fingers. She had been in psychoanalysis for 4 years for this. She was cured rather quickly with a couple of cuts of the surgeon's scalpel as she was suffering from bilateral carpal tunnel syndrome. I asked her how she felt about seeing an analyst for 4 years and spending all that time and she said she was pleased and that it was the best thing that ever happened to her, and she could really enjoy her life to a much fuller extent than she would ever have been able to. Maybe this also applies to marital therapy.

Lila Russell: Can I ask a question about the last slide? You said you stopped the study for ethical reasons because the couples who were getting the cognitive family therapy after 10 sessions were scoring higher on the indexes that you had. Now how does that square with your clinical experience because that's only 10 weeks and I presume in your general clinical work you've seen couples longer than 10 weeks in cognitive family therapy.

Dr. Waring: Now, Ernie mentioned about the ethical business first of all. We started with a different design. We started with the same design as Freidman which was four cells with placebo plus, and as Ernie said, the commonsense of the patients and the staff quickly suggested exactly what he said. It's so self-evident that the antidepressants are effective for major depressions that nobody would participate and when they did, the staff would undermine it whether or not they were getting placebos.

Lila Russell: The staff knew?

Dr. Waring: Well, the staff tried to find out continuously because they felt that the patients weren't getting the treatment that they thought they deserved, so we went to three cells. Cognitive family therapy plus the antidepressant was the study group. Husband and wife together was the control group, having 10 sessions with a psychiatrist. The 10 sessions lasted only 20 minutes. In the third control group, the wife alone saw Dr.

Frelick; she got medication and 20 minutes of supportive individual therapy. Now, don't forget that the prediction was that the antidepressants plus the cognitive family therapy was going to be additive, that it was going to be much better than either of the two control groups. Well, within a total of only 13 patients, which is a very small number, we already had a significant finding of less improvement in the cognitive family therapy group than the two control groups, and the cognitive family therapy group was significantly worse off at 10 weeks. The next question, which Dr. Miles raised in his clinical discussion, is whether cognitive family therapy, not anybody else's marital therapy, just ours, is contraindicated in those individuals with affective disorders who don't get better with the antidepressants alone and in which the combination may be indicated. There certainly may be a group that gets better but still want, at that point in time, marital assessment, and this may prevent further affective disorders. In terms of my clinical experience, I think what you're really suggesting is that in the majority of patients with major affective disorders, the patient in the first session will say, "I feel that I'm not close and can't confide in my spouse." They have a treatment with antidepressant medication so that they are no longer clinically depressed and you say to them, "Do you still want to talk about your dissatisfaction in your marriage?" About 60 percent say, "Did I say that? Did I say there was something wrong with my marriage? I don't remember. I certainly don't feel that way now." So that's my clinical experience with that particular group.

What comes out of the study is a generalization that would be important for us to publish just to say to nonpsychiatrists: When you are screening your clientele for marital therapy you should screen for major affective disorder. You should use a screening instrument if you don't know how to do the history yourself. I think we've all seen couples who have been referred where one or both (it's very common with both) have major affective disorders and have been seeing a counselor for 1, 2, or 3 years and their life has been a living hell. Terrible. And treatment just like the example I gave you of the Chinese couple where treatment of the affective disorder has resulted.

Lila Russell: Where did you get the patients?

Dr. Waring: They were both inpatients and outpatients of this unit but predominantly they were inpatients.

Lila Russell: Yes. And basically weren't they referred as couples?

Dr. Waring: They didn't have to say, "I have a marital problem" to be part of the trial. That's why you have such high dropout rates. It's not a good fit. Controlled outcome studies as Paul mentioned have as many theoretical imperfections to them as do clinical judgments about outcome. For example, the first design resulted in only 20 percent of people with major depressions participating in the study. Well, who were those people? They were people with severe personality disorders and affective disorders. What a group to start testing any hypothesis out on! Then when we switched we got a 50 percent participation rate in this particular study, but again the poor fit is that while a lot of these people said, "Yes, there is some difficulties with the marriage," most of them weren't there for marital therapy in the first place.

Now I'll give you an example of part of the silliness of the controlled trial type of study. I'm seeing one of the control couples now. She's a lady who just had a pregnancy, had a baby, and had a major affective disorder. She has improved clinically so that she is not symptomatic. Part of the study design is that she and her husband with this little infant have to trudge in and see me for 20 minutes once a week and they are tired of coming in. She feels great and they don't have anything to talk about, but if I say, "Don't come back" which is what you would tend to say on clinical grounds, they would be termed a dropout. This is silly since she is feeling well. They would be a dropout if I told them not to come back. Do you understand what I mean? So that although scientifically we talk about controlled studies as being so much better than individual bias, I think the whole issue of therapist bias is overrated. I think most therapists would more honestly evaluate their work if they used a few objective measures. The whole issue is silly. So you get the opposite silliness with this kind of control trial with this couple doing exceptionally well. Any person with commonsense would say, "Don't spend all this time trundling up your 7-week-old infant to come up and say you're still feeling well. Both of you are happy about the way that things turned out."

Lila Russell: It's a nice problem.

Dr. Waring: This is the first of this kind of placebo control research that I have done. It makes me have doubts about all the National Institute of Mental Health patients. Who are these patients who will go in there and go drug-free for a month? It must be the strangest group of individuals in the United States. To put it in perspective, the average woman with a major affective disorder who comes to me as an outpatient and says, "I feel I can't confide in my husband" would receive antidepressant medication. If she didn't have to be hospitalized and came back to see me in two weeks, she would be symptomatically better. I say, "Is there something you want to do about understanding your depression or your relationship?" and as I said, about 50–60 percent say, "No, I don't." So I see her again in another two weeks to make sure the improvement has continued and then refer her back to her family doctor—total therapeutic time about two hours.

Lila Russell: Maybe the one group that is doing sort of combined interventions is the family doctors who are prescribing antidepressants, seeing the couple, maybe asking them, How are things going, how are you doing, maybe seeing the wife when she brings in the baby, and asking her again, How are things going for you. This is very supportive and very facilitating. And again I think maybe these family doctors are the ones who should be doing this sort of research as well.

Dr. Waring: Well, as you probably know, we have talked to the family doctors about doing screening for marital discord, which is the most common place it probably presents, just as you say. People of either sex come in with chronic symptoms, with physical symptoms, chronic tension or minor dysphoria, who want someone they can confide in because they feel that they can't confide in their spouse and I think that this is probably where most marital therapy comes up.

Lila Russell: No more questions.

Dr. Frelick: I would just like to say a few thank-yous, and I'll make this very quick. I'd like to thank Dr. Waring whose idea this meeting was. I'd like to thank the Department of Continuing Education at the University of Western Ontario for the tremendous amount of work they did organizing this conference. I'd like to thank Victoria Hospital and the people in our department for a lot of work. I'd like to thank our sponsors who gave us money to help defray some of the costs. I'd like to thank Peter Martin. I'd like to thank all the people who came such a long way to present papers—Dr. Miles and Dr. Myer from Vancouver, Dr. Guttman from Montreal, Dr. Rosenbluth and Dr. Cameron from Toronto. I'd like to thank all our discussants. Particularly I would like to thank all of you for coming and being involved in this conference for the last 2 days, and on your behalf I would once again thank all the people who presented papers and who participated in the discussions.

Index

Ackerman, N.W., 74
Alexander, J., 114
A Marital Therapy Manual, 8
Analysis, and marital therapy, 25, 26
Alcoholism, 84, 88, 115, 194
Anderson, F.E., 167, 168

Bacal, H., 107
Battle, C., 118
Beavers, W.R., 14
Beck, D.F., 112, 188
Behavioral marital therapy:
  combined therapies, 189, 190
  effectiveness, 105, 108
  techniques, 109
Belsky, J., 171
Bergin, A.E., 106
Berman, E.M., 114
Bowen, M., 74, 75, 81, 112
Bisexuality, 84
Brenner, C., 150, 159
British Medical Journal, 92
Brownell, K.D., 189
Bucher, B., 189

Cameron, P., 59, 111
Candy, J., 120
Claghorn, J.L., 75
Cobb, J.P., 189
Collaborative therapy, 15
  contraindications, 17
  indications for, 17
Complaints, about spouses, *table*, 40
Concurrent therapy, 15, 182, 185
  group, 187, 188
  outcomes, 186, 187
Conjoint marital therapy:
  in combined therapies, 186, 187
  contraindications, 19, 20
  effectiveness, 108
  group, 187–189
  indications, 18, 19
  initial interview, 30–47
    complaints about spouses, 41
    motivation in, 35–37
    variations on, 45, 46
  models of, 15, 16
  for sexual problems, 19
  triadic situations in, 151
Consecutive marital therapy, 15
  contraindications, 18
  indications, 17, 18
Cookerly, J.R., 185, 187–189
Countertransference
  in marital theory, 136–152
  therapist's reactions, 146–149
    child, 147
    parental, 147
    therapeutic strategies, 147–149
Couples therapy, 27
  and combined therapy, 183, 187
  transference in, 138
  triadic situation in, 137
Crowe, M., 109, 112, 114, 117, 119

Davenport, Y.B., 191, 196

Depression:
  in marital therapy clients, 45, 46, 88, 93, 177, 178, 191
  masked, 195
  psychopharmacological treatment, 46, 64, 177, 178, 183, 184, 194, 196–199
Dicks, H.V., 82, 137, 149, 150
Dimascio, D., 120
Divorce therapy, 18, 84
Dove-tailing, 12
Drug therapy, in combined therapies, 183, 184, 191, 194, 196–199
DSM-III, 115, 116

Ely, A.L., 188
Epstein, N., 113
Erickson, M.H., 8, 9
Extramarital affairs, 41, 52, 53, 59, 63, 172
Eysenck, H.J., 106

Family Service of America, 188
Family therapy:
  cognitive, 198
  combined in marital therapy, 190, 191
  conjoint marital therapy in, 14
  creative theories, 8
  dyadic relationships, 137
  joining, 137
  transference in, 136
  triads in, 137
  in combined therapies, 183
Family Therapy, 156
folie à deux, 7, 25
Framo, J.L., 32
Frank., J., 118
Frankel, S., 18
Freeman, S.J., 112
Freud, S., 82, 150, 159
Friedman, A.S., 191, 196, 197, 202
Frude, N., 121

Gale, A., 120
General Health Questionnaire (GHQ), 117

Gestalt therapy, 145
Giovacchini, P.L., 136, 151
Glass, G.V., 107
Glick, I.D., 18
Goldberg, M., 13
Greene, B.L., 137, 151, 182, 183, 185, 196
Grunebaum, H., 59
Gurin, G., 14
Gurman, A., 105, 106, 108, 113, 116, 118, 120, 121, 124, 186, 190
Guttman, H., 113

Hafner, R.J., 189
Haley, J., 7–9, 74, 82, 157
Hartman, L., 111, 124
Hollender, M.H., 12
Hollis, F., 113
Holt, R., 104
Homosexual couples, 14, 24, 84
Hunt, A., 112

Imber, S., 118
Individual marital therapy, 15–17
  concurrent, 15, 182, 185, 187
  consecutive, 15, 17, 18
  contraindications, 17
  countertransference in, 28
  indications, 16
  triangular transference in, 136
Individual therapy, 15, 16, 24, 86–88
  in combined therapies, 183, 185, 187
  contraindications, 16
  indications, 16
  transference and countertransference in, 136, 137
Interpersonal process, 12, 13, 21
Intimacy, 43, 48, 100
Intrapsychic therapy, 11, 12, 21
Interracial or interfaith couples, 84
Isabella, R.A., 171

Jacobson, N.S., 81, 110, 189, 194

Index

Johnson, V., 106, 166
Jones, M., 112
Jung, C.G., 82, 92

Kaplan, H.S., 111, 112, 124
Karasu, T.B., 192
Kessler, D.R., 18
Kireshuk, T., 118
Klein, M., 82
Klerman, G., 120
Kniskern, D., 105, 106, 108, 116, 118, 120, 121, 186
Krueger, D.W., 15
Kupfer, D.J., 168

Laing, R.D., 160
Lambert, M., 106
Lask, B., 121
Leff, J., 191
Levine, J., 75
Liberman, R., 81
Lief, H.I., 114
Locke-Wallace Marital Adjustment Scale, 109
Lumley, P., 112

Malan, D., 107, 118, 120
Marital Interaction Coding System, 109
Marital process, 12-14, 21
  and children, 95, 96
  mismating, 13, 14
Marital therapy:
  analysis in, 20, 25, 26
  antidepressants in, 184
  behavioral, 20, 105, 109
  combined therapies in, 182-200
  concurrent, 15, 182, 185
  conjoint, 14, 16, 18-20, 108, 183
  and drug therapy, 191, 192
  and family therapy, 190, 191
  indications for, 11-22
  motivation for, 35-37
    anger, 62, 63
    assessment of, 56-74
    communication, 66, 67
    factors affecting, 60-65
    goals, 68, 69

sexual problems, 61, 62
specific, 59, 60
outcome research, 104-125
  deterioration rates, 110, 111
  effectiveness, 105-110
  research design, 116-122
overview, 3-10
sexual therapy in, 14, 61, 62, 106, 111, 165-179
techniques of, 83
transference reactions in, 6, 146, 147
types of, 80-94
  behavioral, 81
  psychoanalytic-psychodynamic, 81, 82
Marital Therapy from a Psychiatric Perspective: An Overview, 114
Marks, I., 120
Marriage Contracts and Couple Therapy, 154
Martin, B., 110
Martin, P., 12, 14, 15, 18, 82
Massachusetts General Hospital, 75
Masters, W., 106, 166
McMaster Group, 113, 119
McMaster School of Family Functioning, 133
McMaster University, 75
Mead, M., 5
Mendonca, J., 112
Michels, R., 115
Miles, J., 59
Miller, T.L., 107
Minuchin, S., 28, 74, 81, 144, 157, 161
Mittleman, B., 185

National Institute of Mental Health (NIMH), 117, 205
Nichols, M., 156

Olson's Pair Inventory, 116

Parloff, M.B., 117
Postner, R., 113

Psychopathology, 19, 59, 64, 84, 88, 115
  Alzheimer's disease, 84
  schizophrenia, 66, 84, 176, 194
Psychotherapy:
  effectiveness of, 108–110
  group, 15, 27
  in improvement of marital therapy, 107
  and marital difficulties, 14
  in marital therapy, 9

Rachman, S., 106
Random House College Dictionary, 57
Reid, W.J., 114
Research Diagnostic Criteria, 197
Retaliation:
  husband against wife, *table* 41
  wife against husband, *table* 41
Rosenbluth, M., 111
Ruperstein, C., 167

Sadock, V.A., 15, 18
Sager, C., 14, 82, 105, 154, 167
Santa Barbara, J., 118
Satir, V., 82
Segraves, R.T., 42
Sexual dysfunction, 166–179
  ejaculatory, 167, 172, 175
  erectile, 167, 176
  orgasmic, 167, 172, 175, 178
Sexual therapy:
  and combined therapy, 183
  conjoint treatment in, 19
  effectiveness, 106
  marital assessment, 168–179
  in marital therapy, 14, 111, 112
  relationship to marital therapy, 165–179
Shurman, R., 118

Shyne, A.W., 114
Sifneos, P., 56
Sigal, J., 113
Smith, J.W., 59
Smith, M.L., 107
Solomon, A.P., 137, 151, 182, 183, 185, 196
Spiegel, J., 82
Spouse Observation Check List (SOC), 109
Stuart, R.B., 81
Sullivan, H.S., 82, 150

Transference:
  intervention, methods of, 145, 146
  in marital therapy, 136–152
  nonsexual reactions:
    nonsymmetrical, 139, 140
    symmetrical, 138, 139
  reactions, involvements in, 25
  removal of reactions, 6
  sexualized reactions, 143–146
    heterosexual triangulation, 143–145
    homosexual triangulation, 144, 145
  therapeutic strategies, 140–142
  triangular, 136–138

University of Michigan, 6

Victoria Hospital, 13

Waring's Intimacy Questionnaire, 116
Walrond-Skinner, S., 14, 20
Wattie, B., 112
Weisz, G.M., 189
Whitaker, C., 9, 78
Wolberg, L., 79
Woodward, C., 118, 119